MODERN TECHNIQUES
OF ACUPUNCTURE
Volume II

A critical review of European developments
in acupuncture.

By the same author:
ACUPRESSURE TECHNIQUES
CLINICAL ECOLOGY *with Dr George Lewith*
MODERN TECHNIQUES OF ACUPUNCTURE Volume I
MODERN TECHNIQUES OF ACUPUNCTURE Volume III
TWENTY FIRST CENTURY MEDICINE

MODERN TECHNIQUES OF ACUPUNCTURE

A practical scientific guide to electronic pulsography, auriculotherapy and neural therapy

Volume II

by
JULIAN N. KENYON
M.D., M.B., Ch.B.

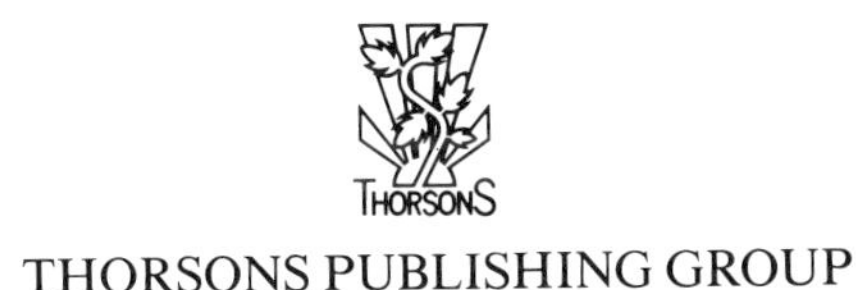

THORSONS PUBLISHING GROUP

First published 1983

British Library Cataloguing in Publication Data

Kenyon, Julian N.
Modern techniques of acupuncture.
Vol. 2: A practical scientific guide to electro-acupuncture
1. Acupuncture
I. Title
615.8'92   RM184

ISBN 0-7225-0751-8

*Published by Thorsons Publishers Limited,
Wellingborough, Northamptonshire, NN8 2RQ, England*

Printed in Great Britain by Woolnough Bookbinding Limited,
Irthlingborough, Northamptonshire

3   5   7   9   10   8   6   4

CONTENTS

DEDICATION

To Margaret

INTRODUCTION

Volume II follows the format set out in Volume I in that a practical guide is given together with important references to new fields of acupuncture.

The first section of the book looks at electronic pulsography, that is the recording of the traditional Chinese pulse using piezo-electric transducers with the recording of the pulse characteristics on an oscilloscope. This represents the only new technique within acupuncture which records a totally traditional Chinese concept: that of the Chinese pulse. The observation that the pulse shapes recorded are entirely consistent with those predicted by the ancient Chinese originators of acupuncture perhaps raises more questions than answers. The consistency of pulse recording taken from the same patient on consecutive days is an impressive feature, and the use of the law of the five elements as seemingly the only way to alter the recording, must be important observations. At the time of writing no trials or in depth studies of the traditional Chinese pulse have appeared. As interest in acupuncture by the Western medical profession increases, investigation of the findings of electronic pulsography will become an important new area of research. It would be wrong to reject these findings simply because they appear strange and inexplicable.

The second section of this book deals with auricular therapy and auricular medicine, as developed by the French school, led by Dr Paul Nogier. Auricular therapy is a simple technique which revolves around the detection of tender points on the auricle. To date no authritative account of this method has appeared.

Auricular medicine is a sophistication of auricular therapy, based upon the auricular cardiac reflex as a basic biological measure. Of all the developments within modern acupuncture the auricular cardiac reflex remains the most difficult to record. It is not clear why this should be so, but this difficulty has given rise to considerable controversy surrounding the whole discipline of auricular medicine. It does, however, represent a legitimate new area of therapy which has so far not been written about in the English language.

Auricular medicine naturally leads on to the more forward looking therapeutic techniques which have emerged from acupuncture; that is the use of lasers and magnetic fields. The literature on the use of lasers is very sparse indeed and must therefore be looked upon with some scepticism for the time being, but in practice lasers remain useful therapeutic tools.

The use of magnetic fields in therapy, has, in contrast, more solid scientific backing. Indeed, so much so that a separate chapter has been devoted to an up-to-date survey of the biological effects of magnetic fields. The perceptive reader will gather that the disciplines of physics and electronics are going to be as important as that of medicine in the further investigation and development of these new fields.

This book, like Volume I, is designed to satisfy the therapist and the academic alike. The therapist is recommended to learn the simple techniques first and apply them in practice before going on to more advanced techniques. As appropriate research is carried out, then some of the disciplines in this book may well be discarded, as others will be developed. This is inevitable in a new field which has as yet received less than its fair share of attention from academic medicine. A critical approach is therefore important to all of the techniques outlined in this volume.

Those doctors wishing to master electronic pulsography or auricular therapy/medicine, are advised to try to attend appropriate training courses, a number of which are available worldwide.

HOW TO USE THIS BOOK

The book is divided into two volumes; the first volume deals with electro-acupuncture and neuro-electric therapy, and finishes with a section on electro-acupuncture according to Voll. Volume II deals with electronic pulsography and then goes on to auricular therapy, finishing with a section on aricular medicine.

Each section is complete in itself and may be used as such. It is recommended that practitioners should read both volumes to get a general idea of what is available, and then choose one topic to learn thoroughly. Auricular therapy is the simplest and the easiest to practice, and this should be the first discipline which any practitioner new to these areas of acupuncture should approach.

Each section begins with basic concepts and becomes gradually more complex. It is possible to learn each method in parts; in other words in the case of auricular therapy and auricular medicine, it is possible to learn auricular therapy and put it into practice, and on having gained competence in auricular therapy, the next logical step would be to learn the auricular cardiac reflex and go on to apply the more sophisticated ideas of auricular medicine. In the same way with electro-acupuncture according to Voll, it is possible to learn the basic concepts and then to measure points on a number of patients in order to get used to defining the pathology in EAV terms. It is not necessary to come to grips immediately with homoeopathic medicine testing, which is a very complex subject itself.

In the author's view, it is not possible to gain competence at any of the disciplines discussed in this book without practical training, and to this end the author devotes much of his time to running training courses in the practical aspects of the branches of acupuncture discussed here.

Throughout both volumes, protocols have been outlined and these are designed for use with the patient in a clinical situation. It is envisaged that practitioners starting to learn any one of the subjects discussed in this book will begin by reading the section a number of times, and then by working with patients with the relevant page of the book open at the appropriate protocol. The same applies to the photographs and line drawings, in particular the charts which accompany the text, for example, in 'Electro-acupuncture according to Voll' the charts are specifically designed for than fifty per cent of the information contained in the pulsograph. In the author's opinion this observation must have practical implications for those teaching acupuncture.

History At the time of the *Nei Ching Su Wen* (250 BC) the pulses of the different organs were palpated on different parts of the body rather than on the radial pulse. To judge the energy in any meridian particular points were palpated and all of these points lay over palpable arteries. For example, Liver 3 was palpated to ascertain liver energy; Kidney 3 for kidney energy; Spleen 11 for spleen energy; Lung 8 for lung energy etc. These were the forerunners of traditional pulse diagnosis as we know it today.

Pien Chhio (pronounced Pen Chow) is regarded as the father of traditional pulse diagnosis. Pien Chhio wrote the *Nan Ching*. The exact date of the *Nan Ching* (not to be confused with the *Nei Ching*) is unknown, as is the date of Pien Chhio himself. However, it can be said that the *Nan Ching* was published at least 200 BC. The *Nan Ching* is also sometimes referred to as *The Pulse Book of Pien Chhio*. In this book the pulses of the four seasons are described, and in Chapters 2 and 17 the exact location of the pulse palpation points and organ correspondence of these points was shown for the first time.

Pien Chhio became famous in China and a number of stories relate to him. One of particular relevance is the advice Pien Chhio gave to King Huan. Pien Chhio felt the King's pulse and said that the king had a disease on the skin and that he needed treatment. The King was angry at this and sent Pien Chhio away. Five days later Pien Chhio returned and requested a further audience with the King, and again he felt his pulse. He told the King that he now had a disease of the blood and that the disease process was becoming more deeply situated. Pien Chhio advised the King that he needed treatment, but again the King was angry and sent Pien Chhio away. Pien Chhio returned for a third time, after a lapse of a few days, and asked for a further audience with the King. Again, he felt his pulse, and said that the King now had a disease in the intestines and the liver, and that the King needed treatment. The King responded in the same way and Pien Chhio was again sent away. Pien Chhio returned a fourth time, but this time ran away from the King. Following this, King Huan called for him and asked why he had run away. Pien Chhio told the King that he now had a disease of the marrow which cannot be treated. Pien Chhio told the King that a disease on the skin can be treated with wrappings; a disease in the blood can be treated with acupuncture and moxibustion; diseases in the organs can be treated with herbs, but a disease in the marrow cannot be treated. Pien Chhio then left the King. After a few weeks the King fell seriously ill and the Imperial Court sent out messengers to find Pien Chhio to ask him to come to treat the King. Pien Chhio couldn't be found and the King died soon after.

This story shows that Pien Chhio's expertise was due in large measure to his ability to palpate the pulse and derive useful information from it. He also recognized that different forms of treatment were necessary depending on how deep the pathology had got. It is interesting to note his comment that the treatment of disease which had reached the organs was best done by herbs. This is effectively the equivalent of homoeopathy in our present system of medical care, and it is fascinating to reflect that the findings of EAV and medicine testing substantiate Pien Chhio's advice.

Many other later books were written on the traditional pulse, culminating in a number of compendiums published in the sixteenth century. The text used by D. J. Yoo in order to interpret the pulsograph is the *Tongi Bo Gan* ('Treatise of Eastern Medicine') by Hue Jun. It was published in 1613. This book combines all of Eastern medicine and deals with the pulse diagnosis in a detailed manner.

The Traditional Chinese Pulse

Traditional Chinese medicine holds that on the radial pulse on each hand there are three positions; each of these three positions being further sub-divided into a superficial and deep level. The middle position lies immediately adjacent to the radial styloid process on each side. The proximal position lies one finger's breadth proximal to the radial styloid process, and the distal position lies one finger's breadth distal to the same process. This is illustrated in Figure 1.

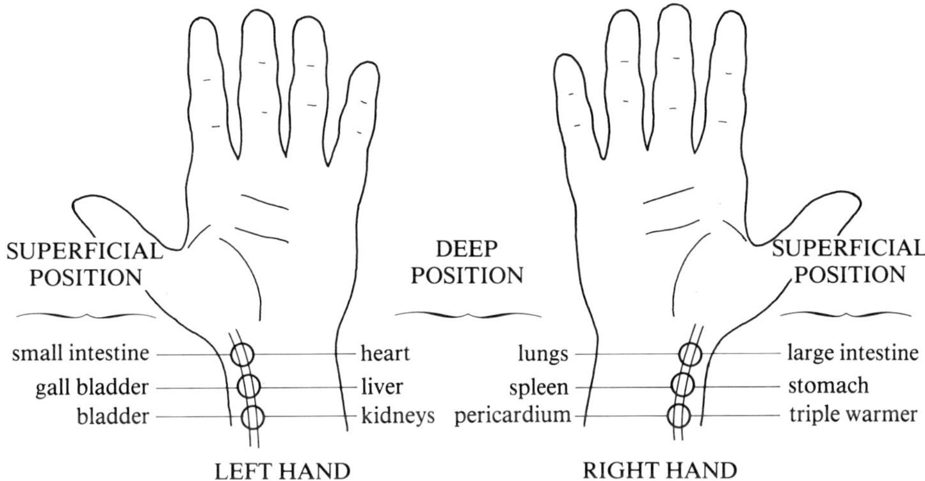

Figure 1.   Positions of the pulse diagnosis.

The pulse at each position was thought to correspond to the meridians as indicated. The suggestion that by feeling one part of the radial pulse the state of health of a remote organ can be ascertained is preposterous enough, and the possibility that pulse shapes recorded from areas on one artery lying within a few centimeters of each other can be in any significant degree different, is very hard to accept. The fact that these phenomena can now be recorded using the equipment developed by Drs Yoo and Paik probably raises more questions than answers.

Traditional Chinese Ideas and the Pulse

Traditional Chinese medicine does not regard the traditional pulse, as here described, as being a vessel wall phenomenon alone, and it regards the blood inside the blood vessel as being of greater importance than the vessel wall. In order to understand this it is necessary to have a broad understanding of Chinese ideas of blood and energy (chi). Unfortunately there is no way of incorporating these ancient conceptual paradigms into terms of modern science, therefore in order for the pulse recordings to be useful it is necessary to understand something of traditional Chinese bio-energetics. This suggestion is often greeted with reluctance on the part of many Western practitioners, and many therefore do not even attempt to understand the system in depth, as, for example, excellently explained by Porkert.[1] This reluctance is summarized by a passage in *Celestial Lancets*, by Needham and Lu, page 185.[2] In it a French practitioner is quoted as stressing the danger of applying modern concepts of energy to classical Chinese ideas of energy (chi), and especially with regard to the many facile analogies with biophysical electric currents etc. This is a statement with which the author whole-heartedly agrees. However, he goes on to say:

> The yin and yang were intrinsically pre-renaissance ideas, in that they could be made to explain anything, and the five elements are as unacceptable today as Aristotle's four — yet, in spite of this, many Western physicians practising acupuncture, showed an 'illuminisme' which has no need of laboratory tests or modern diagnostic procedures. If we wish to be taken seriously, and not to be confused with bone setters and faith healers, we must abandon the whole more or less Chinese mass of philosophy, cosmogony, and mythology in which we have been entangled these forty years past. Let us clear the decks and look at our problems without preconceived ideas. The study of the anatomy and physiology of the skin, and of the central and sympathetic nervous systems, the investigation of the physico-chemical and enzymic reactions in the body, all these should provide us with a means of solving the problem of what acupuncture really is and does.

Similar sentiments have been expressed by doctors, and indeed many of them practitioners of acupuncture throughout the world. In the author's view the findings of electronic pulsography, and those of EAV should make us stop and think again. It is interesting to note the comments of Needham and Lu with regard to the above quote. Their comment is as follows:

> Though a rather extreme statement, this has the interest of coming from a Western acupuncture physician, and many of his colleagues in China would agree with him. For ourselves, we retain reservations.

Traditional Chinese medicine often couples blood (hsueh) and energy (chi) together. Blood (hsueh) is thought to be produced and stored in the middle heater; that is essentially the stomach, spleen and liver from where it is distributed throughout the body, in accordance with demand. The Ling-Shu states that 'blood (hsueh) and chi are different in name, yet similar in kind.' Chi is regarded as yang, and blood is regarded as yin. Yoo states[3] that the pulse is a result of interplay of these two energies; yin (inside, and synonymous with blood) and yang (outside and synonymous with chi). The explanation given here is simplistic in comparison to that given by Porkert.[1] However, it serves to explain the concept and interested readers should consult Porkert's book.

As the pulsograph recording is a recording of a traditional Chinese concept its interpretation has to be made within the same paradigm, otherwise no practical sense can be made out of the recording. This will become apparent when interpretation of pulse shapes and appropriate treatment, together with clinical examples are given. The treatment based on pulsography is therefore determined according to the law of the five elements (Wu Hsing).

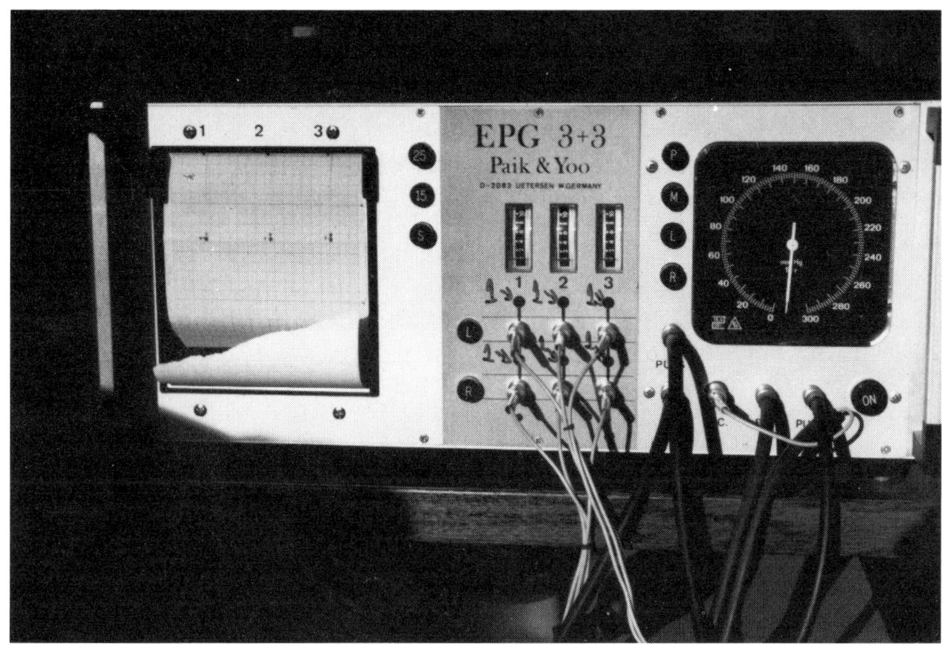

Figure 2a.   EPG unit showing paper recorder.

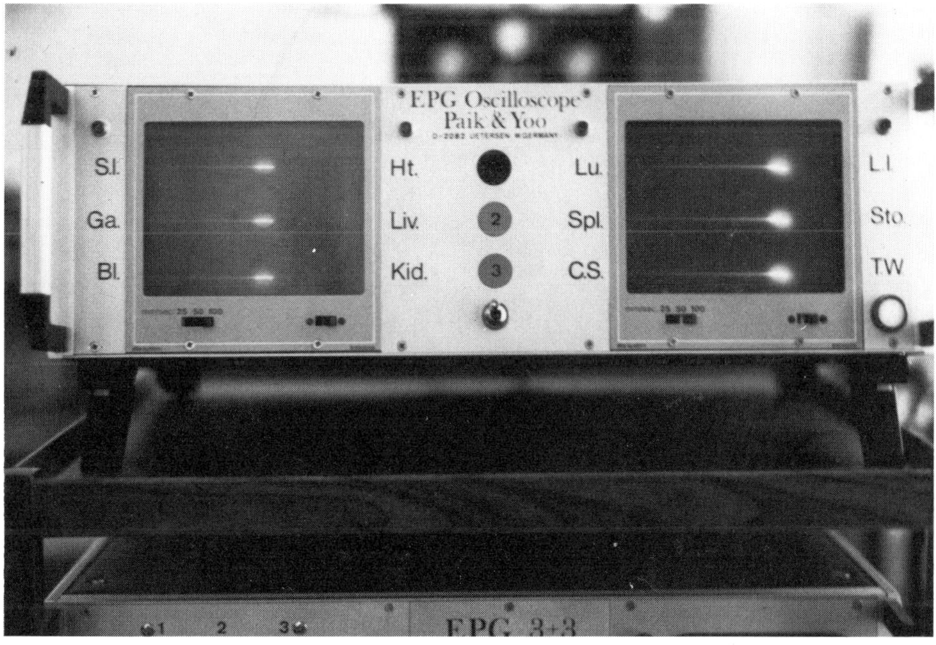

Figure 2b.   EPG unit showing continuous readout unit.

Equipment The electronic pulsograph consists of six piezo-electric pulse transducers, colour coded red, yellow and blue corresponding to distal, middle and proximal pulse palpation points on each side. The transducers are connected to a recording device with an ECG type paper recording strip for recording input from three transducers on one side simultaneously. The right-hand side of this unit has a sphygmomanometer pressure gauge which can be switched either to a blood pressure recording cuff which contains a microphone for electronic recording of blood pressure, or to either right- or left-sided inflatable rubber cuffs for wrapping round each wrist to keep the transducers in position. This represents the basic unit, and is illustrated in Figures 2a, 2b and 3.

An accessory unit is available which has a six channel continuous oscilloscope readout, three channels on the left and three on the right. This can be connected into the main unit. This accessory unit is not an essential part of the pulsograph equipment but it is useful for those practitioners wishing to see pulse changes happening during treatment as it enables them to try various point combinations, and to see what, if any, immediate effects are produced. This is illustrated in Figures 2a and 2b.

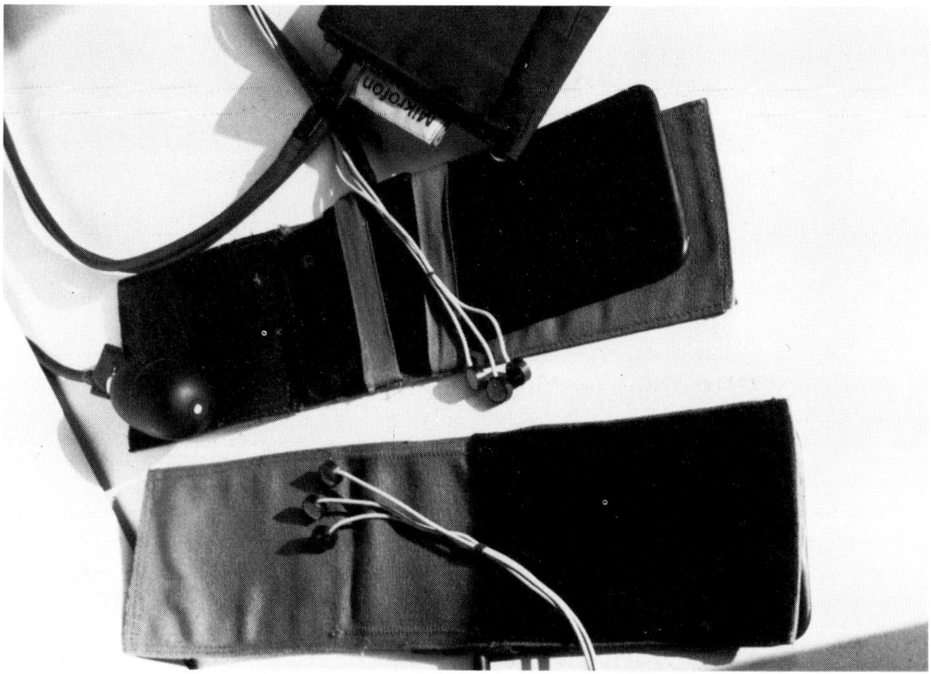

Figure 3.   Pulse transducers and cuffs for use with the EPG.

Method of Pulse 1. Measure blood pressure on right and left arm, using either the blood pressure
Recording Using   cuffs supplied with the pulsograph together with the microphone and electronic
the Pulsograph   blood pressure readout, or take with a manual sphygmomanometer. This is
                           the author's practice as he finds it quicker and regards the automatic blood
                           pressure recording side of the pulsograph as an unnecessary addition to the
                           equipment.

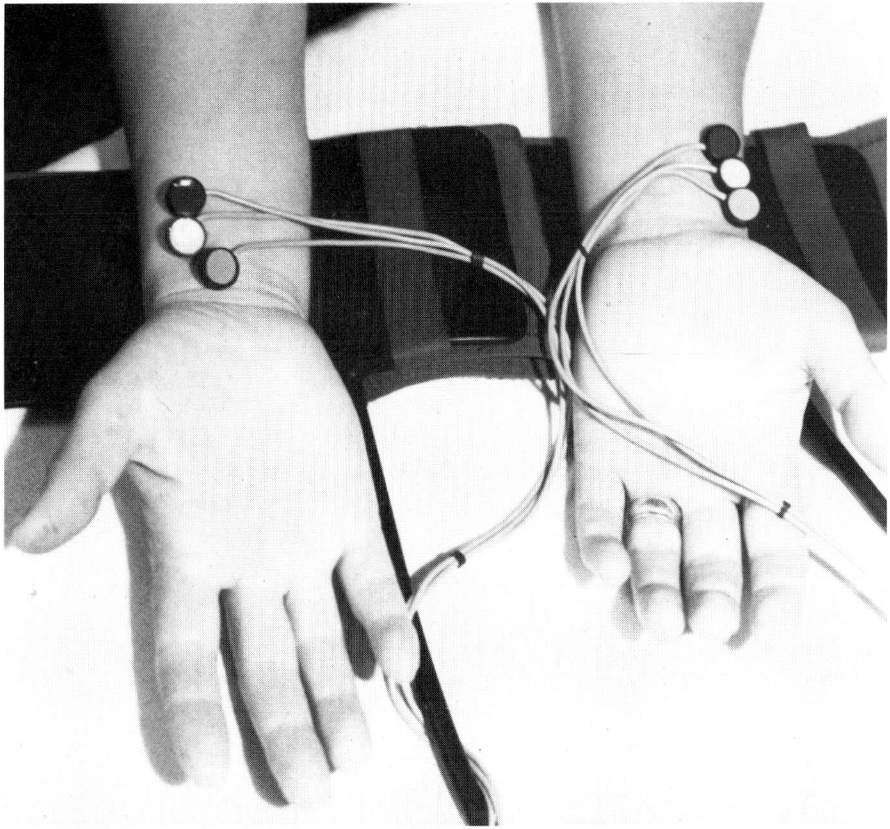

Figure 4.   Applying the pulse transducers to the pulse.

2. Extend both wrists with the appropriate pulse cuff beneath each wrist, and apply
    the pulse transducers in the correct sequence (red, yellow, blue). Apply with
    the colour side uppermost and the convex side of the transducer against the
    pulse. This is illustrated in Figure 4.
3. Carefully wrap the pulse cuff around each wrist, taking care not to disturb the
    positions of the pulse transducers (Figures 5 and 6).
4. Inflate either the right or left pulse cuff with the appropriate switches depressed
    on the main unit of the EPG, up to diastolic pressure plus 5 millimeters of
    Mercury. This corresponds to the superficial pulse pressure at which level the
    pulses of the hollow (fu) organs are recorded (Large Intestine, Stomach, Triple
    Warmer on the right side; Small Intestine, Gall Bladder and Bladder on the
    left side).
5. Press recording button for paper recording of pulse.
6. Inflate the same pulse cuff up to systolic blood pressure minus 5 millimeters
    of Mercury. This corresponds to the deep pulse pressure, and at this pressure
    the pulses of the solid (zang) organs are recorded (Lung, Spleen, Pericardium
    on the right side; Heart, Liver and Kidney on the left side).
7. Press paper recording button and record the deep pulses.
8. Deflate cuff on side measured. Follow exactly the same procedure for the

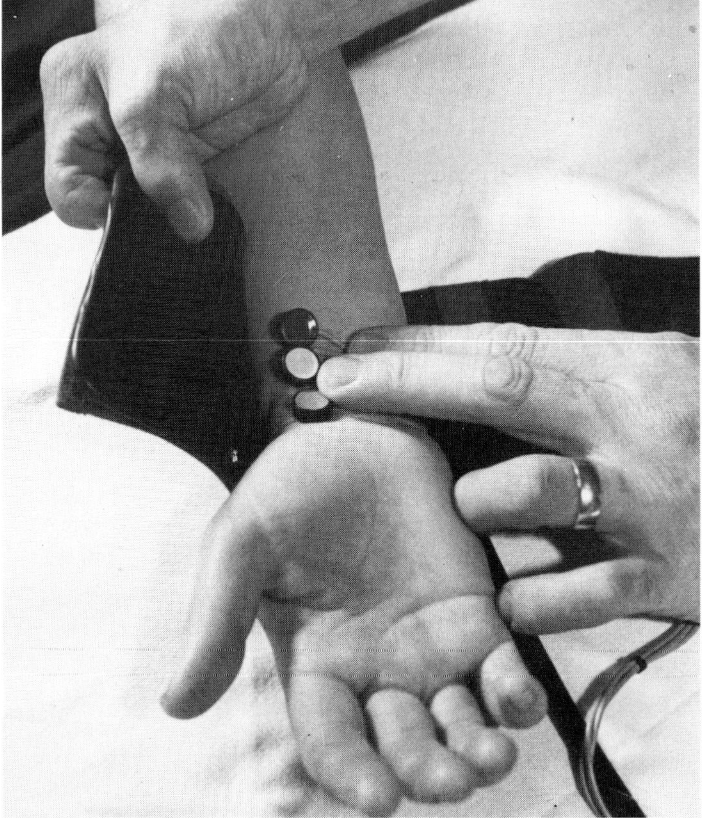

Figure 5.   Wrapping up pulse cuff around the wrist over the transducers.

opposite side. If a continuous readout is required of either the superficial or the deep organs then the pulse cuff will have to remain inflated at either diastolic plus 5mm Mercury (for the superficial organs), or at systolic pressure minus 5mm Mercury (for the deep organs). Then treatment can proceed whilst observing any changes in the pulse.

Calibration of the Pulsograph   It is important that each transducer, if subjected to the same pulse pressure, should record the same deviation on the tracing as any of the other pulse transducers. The pulse transducers are essentially recording pressure waves. The procedure for calibrating the equipment is as follows, and this should be checked at least every six months. (In the author's experience the pulse transducers aren't always exactly equal in sensitivity, and they are prone to damage, so care is required in handling.)

1. Apply one pulse transducer over one wrist, and attach the cuff around this transducer. Inflate to diastolic pressure plus 5mm Mercury. Plug into each jack plug socket, labelled 1, 2 and 3 left and right on the EPG main unit. A more or less equal deflection of the recording pen should be recorded for each channel.
2. If a channel is recording less than the amplitude of the other channels, then

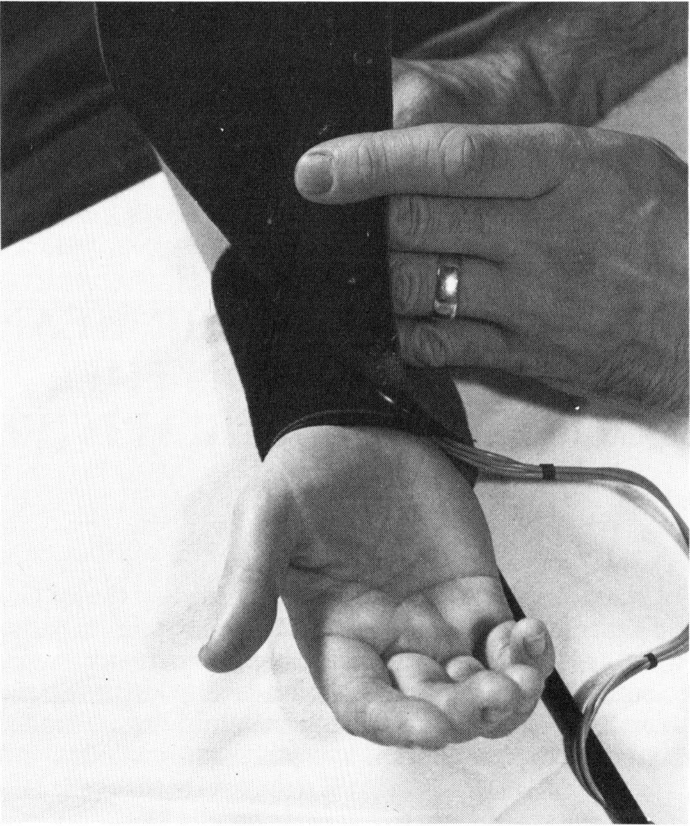

Figure 6. Pulse cuffs wrapped around the wrists ready for recording.

the adjusting screw, lying directly above each jack plug socket, should be turned in a clockwise direction to increase the amplitude of recording. If the recording is too high then this screw should be turned in an anti-clockwise direction.
3. Check each pulse transducer separately on the same pulse measurement point, and check that a more or less equal amplitude is being recorded. If any particular transducer is recording too high or too low then the sensitivity screw on that particular channel relative to the transducer which is recording abnormally, will have to be permanently set, either to reduce or to increase its channel sensitivity, depending on whether the transducer is recording too high or too low. It is not common to find transducers to be grossly out of balance with each other, but this is worth checking as if the machine is not properly calibrated the validity of the recording is not as reliable.

Summary

An introduction to electronic pulsography is given, together with a history of traditional Chinese concepts surrounding the traditional Chinese pulse. An explanation of the necessity for a traditional Chinese explanation of the pulsograph is given.

The equipment is described together with a protocol for pulse recording and for calibrating the equipment.

of the phase preceeding, will tonify that phase; in other words, it will move the cycle round one, whereas stimulating the phase after the evolutive phase under consideration will sedate this phase. Therefore, in terms of the mother/son law* tonifying the mother produces tonification of the son, and stimulation of the son

TABLE 2

1.	Wood	Liver and Gall Bladder
2.	Fire	Heart and Small Intestine Pericardium and Triple Warmer
3.	Earth	Spleen and Stomach
4.	Metal	Lungs and Large Intestine
5.	Water	Kidney and Bladder

TABLE 3

	Tonification Points	*Sedation Points*
Liver	Liver 8	Liver 2
Gall Bladder	Gall Bladder 43	Gall Bladder 38
Heart	Heart 9	Heart 7
Small Intestine	Small Intestine 3	Small Intestine 8
Pericardium	Pericardium 9	Pericardium 7
Triple Warmer	Triple Warmer 3	Triple Warmer 10
Spleen	Spleen 2	Spleen 5
Stomach	Stomach 41	Stomach 45
Lung	Lung 9	Lung 5
Large Intestine	Large Intestine 11	Large Intestine 2
Kidney	Kidney 7	Kidney 1
Urinary Bladder	Urinary Bladder 67	Urinary Bladder 65

* Mother/son law is the same as the production (sometimes called creating) sequence.

gives sedation of the mother. As an example, take the evolutive phase Wood; in order to tonify Wood, Water would be tonified (in this case, Water is the mother of Wood). In order to sedate Wood, Fire would be stimulated (Fire is the son of Wood in this particular case). All of the above is contained in Figure 39.

To each evolutive phase, a pathogen is assigned, i.e. Wind to Wood; Heat to Fire; Damp to Earth; Dryness to Metal; Cold to Water. A five element designation is also given to each meridian pair as in Table 2.

It can be seen from Table 3, that all the tonification and sedation points are worked out according to the mother/son law; that is in keeping with the production sequence, sometimes called 'creating cycle' of the five evolutive phases (Hsing-Sheng-Hsu).

TABLE OF POINTS ACCORDING TO THE FIVE EVOLUTIVE PHASES

Yin Meridians:

Organ	Element	Wood	Fire	Earth	Metal	Water
Lung	Metal	Lu11	Lu10	Lu9	Lu8	Lu5
Heart	Fire	He9	He8	He7	He4	He3
Pericardium	Fire	Pc9	Pc8	Pc7	Pc5	Pc3
Liver	Wood	Liv1	Liv2	Liv3	Liv4	Liv8
Spleen	Earth	Sp1	Sp2	Sp3	Sp5	Sp9
Kidney	Water	Ki1	Ki2	Ki5	Ki7	Ki10

Yang Meridians:

Organ	Element	Metal	Water	Wood	Fire	Earth
Large Intestine	Metal	LI1	LI2	LI3	LI5	LI11
Small Intestine	Fire	SI1	SI2	SI3	SI5	SI8
Triple Warmer	Fire	TW1	TW2	TW3	TW6	TW10
Gall Bladder	Wood	GB44	GB43	GB41	GB38	GB34
Stomach	Earth	St45	St44	St43	St41	St36
Bladder	Water	BL67	BL66	BL65	BL60	BL54

Interpretation of Electronic Pulsographs (EPGs) Based on the Theory of the Five Evolutive Phases

In general, the situation shown on an EPG indicates one pathogen invading a number of meridians; it is unusual to have more than one pathogen present, but this is possible. For example, pathogens cold and heat can co-exist in the same EPG (see examples). Also situations of energy deficiency, energy excess and energy accumulation are shown.

The first observation on looking at a pulsograph is that the recordings from each pulse position are generally different. In many cases these differences are obvious, even to the untrained observer. The differences in pulse shapes from the superficial to the deep position at each pulse measurement point, are never as marked as the differences between the recordings obtained at the individual pulse palpation points, and indeed, the recordings on these superficial and deep levels are often similar, but can again be different, and examples are shown of such differences (see later). In traditional Chinese terms, and from the point of view of treatment, this must be taken as indicating the close functional connection between organ pairs, as laid out on the pulse palpation points. After noting the above general observations a suggested method for reading EPGs is as follows:

1. Look for any situation of excess energy in any particular meridian. If this is grossly in excess in relationship to all other recordings, then it is likely that this is so-called violation or aggressive energy (also known as redundant energy, see table 1). The importance of recognizing redundant or aggressive energy is that it is possible that this energy may trigger the so-called violation sequence of the five evolutive phases. This is a pathological sequence and will have to be dealt with first, before any other therapy in terms of acupuncture can be expected to work. The violation sequence is the K'o cycle in reverse order, as wood violates metal; metal violates fire; fire violates water; water violates earth, and earth in turn violates wood (see Figure 39).

2. If aggressive energy is present, then disperse it. The following example will clarify this. If the position wood (i.e. the liver or gall bladder meridian on the EPG) has an EPG reading of energy excess, and no other meridian shows such energy excess, at least to the degree recorded on the liver or gall bladder meridian, then this energy (wood) will no longer simply check the quality of earth (via the K'o cycle, see Figure 39), but will encroach on it; in other words, it will overcheck and will damage earth. It will also violate metal according to the violation sequence (that is the K'o cycle in reverse) which, according to the K'o cycle, should check wood. However, the violation sequence has reversed this, therefore aggressive or redundant energy leads both to a violation sequence and an exaggerated K'o or checking sequence.

   The treatment is to disperse wood; that is the liver meridian, by sedating it, using Liver 2 (see table of points). It is also necessary to tonify earth as it is under attack from an exaggerated checking (K'o cycle) sequence, therefore the earth meridian, either spleen or stomach, should be tonified. It is sensible that if the liver meridian is the meridian affected with aggressive energy, and as this meridian represents a yin organ, then similarly yin organs should be chosen for treatment. Conversely, if the gall bladder meridian was the meridian largely affected by aggressive energy, and this is a yang organ, then similarly yang organs should be chosen for treatment. Therefore, either Spleen 2 in the case of the liver meridian affected by aggressive energy, or Stomach 41 in the case of the gall bladder meridian being affected by aggressive energy should be used.

Stimulating the element earth has the effect of tonifying metal according to the creating cycle of the five evolutive phases, as laid out in the mother/son law. This will therefore protect metal from being violated by the aggressive energy in wood.

3. If no aggressive energy is present then the pathogen involved should be identified by classifying it into one of the pulse shapes, as outlined in the previous chapter (i.e. wind, heat, damp, dryness and cold). Remember that the scattered pulse from extreme dryness is often difficult to differentiate from a pulse recording due to the pathogen heat. The differences are that with the pathogen heat the peaks tend to be rounded, and of greater amplitude than the peaks recorded from a scattered pulse in the case of extreme dryness. Conversely the peaks in extreme dryness tend to be sharp pointed. Recognizing a damp pulse recording can be very difficult indeed as the characteristics of a damp recording are a wide complex, and often it is a matter of opinion as to whether a complex is widened or not. The author's practice in these cases is to also rely on clinical information from the patient's history, for example, a disease in which the pathogen damp may be involved, such as in ulcerative colitis or chronic bronchitis, or if the tongue diagnosis shows an obvious indication of damp such as a greasy tongue coating, then this would raise the practitioner's suspicion of the pathogen damp on the recording, even though otherwise, without this information, it might not be so obvious.

4. Give each pathogen an identity from one of the five evolutive phases, i.e. wind corresponds to wood; heat corresponds to fire, etc. (see Figure 39).

5. Choose the meridian which is most markedly affected, and disperse the pathogen in that meridian, according to the five evolutive phases using the mother/son law, for example, if wind (wood in the five evolutive phases) is affecting the liver meridian, then this ought to be dispersed by sedating wood, which in the liver meridian is achieved by stimulating the fire point (Liver 2).

6. If the pathogen is affecting both organs of an organ pair, then decide as to whether the condition is a largely yang condition, or a yin condition; for example, a largely yang condition will show most abnormalities above the zero line, and will tend to be present when yang pathogens are invading, such as wind, heat etc. Conversely, a largely yin condition will be manifested by an invasion of yin pathogen such as cold and damp etc. In the case of a largely yin condition then the superficial or yang organ of the organ pair (the Fu organ) should be chosen throughout treatment, conversely, if the condition is largely yang, then yin organs should be chosen from each pair. If this system has not produced a change in the pulsograph when the patient returns on a subsequent appointment, then reverse one's method of treatment and use yang meridians only in yang conditions, and vice versa. It is important to try single ideas out in therapy with the EPG, without mixing them with other ideas at each clinical session, so that as clear a picture as possible evolves and so that only a few ideas in terms of acupuncture therapy are applied with each selection of points.

7. If any evolutive phase is deficient in energy this should be treated at the same time as dispersing the pathogen, simply by tonifying the evolutive phase involved. For example, if the spleen meridian (earth) shows energy defifiency, then this can be tonified via the tonification point on the spleen meridian (Spleen

2). If earth is deficient in energy it would be more easily checked via the K'o cycle by wood; this would have the effect of overchecking it, and therefore making it even more deficient in energy. So this has to be countered by strengthening earth, i.e. by tonifying the spleen via Spleen 2.

There is also a possibility that a violation sequence may arise from the element water; not that the element water in this case contains aggressive energy, but in relationship to the deficiency of energy in the earth meridian the relative energy excess in the water evolutive phase may result in a violation sequence building up, which will further tend to reduce the energy in the earth meridian (spleen). Therefore if Spleen 2 has not produced a change in the EPG, the tonification point on the liver meridian (wood) could be used, which according to the mother/son law would have the effect of sedating the evolutive phase water (in this case, wood, i.e. liver, is the son of water). This will have the effect of minimizing any chance of a violation sequence building up via water in the direction of earth.

8. If on subsequent appointments the EPG has not changed towards normality, then choose another method of point selection according to the five evolutive phases.

9. If the EPG shows the pathogen cold, use moxa either on back shu points, or on front mu points in alternation, or on back shu points alone.

Protocol
1. Identify aggressive energy and disperse if present.
2. Identify pathogen (in some cases, pathogens) invading.
3. Disperse the pathogen (in some cases, pathogens) in the meridian or meridians most obviously affected. Do this by giving the pathogen an identity in the five evolutive phase cycle, and in order to disperse it tonify the evolutive phase point, which is the next point occurring in a clockwise direction from the evolutive phase identity of the pathogen, i.e. to disperse the pathogen wind (wood) in any particular meridian use the fire point on that same meridian.
4. Tonify any energy deficient meridian either by the tonification point on that meridian, and/or sedating the evolutive phase which may be violating the energy deficient meridian using the mother/son law (example given above).

   Another way of sedating the evolutive phase which may be violating the deficient meridian is to use a point sedating that evolutive phase on the energy deficient meridian itself, as well as using the tonification point on the same meridian; this represents another possibility for treating energy deficiency.
5. If the pathogen cold is indicated on the EPG then this must be treated with moxa, and this is best accomplished using moxa on the appropriate back shu points. Front mu points may also be used in alternation with back shu points, although the author prefers to use back shu points alone and is in the habit of giving the patient a moxa stick, and instructing a relative on the application of moxa on the appropriate sites on a daily basis. For further details of moxibustion see *Modern Chinese Acupuncture*.[5] If the pathogen cold has penetrated deeply (see explanation of EPG pulse shapes), then in the author's opinion moxibustion is essential. If cold has only penetrated superficially then needling may be adequate in righting the situation.

   It is obvious from the foregoing that there are a number of methods available for treating any particular situation recorded by an EPG. For example, another method of treating energy excess is to use the Luo or connecting point on the coupled meridian, and drain the energy off via the secondary meridian which joins the coupled organ at the Luo connecting point. (For a list of Luo connecting points, see *Essentials of Chinese Acupuncture*, (1980), published by Foreign Language Press, Peking.)

The most important principle to adhere to is to be sensible and systematic, and only use one law at a time when one is treating using the EPG, otherwise confusion will result. The interrelationships of traditional medicine are very complex but in order to realize their benefit they must be applied in a reasoned way, and the EPG offers a golden opportunity to do this. A number of examples are given in the next chapter to illustrate some of the above rules.

Summary

The law of the five evolutive phases is outlined in detail together with the three cycles of the evolutive phases; two physiological (the creating, or Sheng cycle, and the checking, or K'o cycle), and one pathological (the so-called violation sequence).

The interpretation of the EPG is explained and the treatment based on the EPG, using the rules contained in the five evolutive phases and its cycles are explained in detail.

A protocol for doing this is given, both in a long, and in an abbreviated form.

CHAPTER FOUR

CLINICAL EXAMPLES OF EPGs AND THEIR INTERPRETATION

Ten clinical examples of EPGs are illustrated together with a choice of acupuncture points used on these patients, and an explanation given for the choice of these points. All of the clinical examples given are of patients who have not responded to acupuncture based on a selection of points made after a clinical traditional Chinese diagnosis. All of the patients responded to acupuncture therapy after having made a choice of points based on the pulsograph; this is a common occurrence in the author's practice and it is suggested that firstly, the choice of acupuncture points in any particular patient is important, as only particular sets of points seem to have a therapeutic effect in particular patients; secondly, that electronic pulsography is a useful diagnostic tool as in most cases it leads to more effective therapy in terms of acupuncture, and lastly, the five evolutive phases and the accompanying rules and interrelations of each phase probably ought to be taken more seriously and subjected to further investigation.

The electronic pulsograph renders further investigation of these traditional Chinese theories a practical possibility.

When working through the clinical examples the Five Element diagram (Figure 39) and the list of points referrable to each phase (Table 4) should be constantly referred to.

Normal Pulsographs A Normal pulsograph has not been seen or recorded by the author. The features to look for on a 'normal' pulsograph are that each recording representing each meridian should have an approximately equal positive and negative deflection. There should be no gross imbalances in amplitude between any of the recordings. Gross in this case means the largest deflection being no greater than approximately three times the smallest deflection as recorded respectively on the meridian with the most energy present at the time of recording, and the meridian with the least energy present at the time of recording. Also there should be no wave form indicative of any of the pathogens as indicated in the section on 'wave forms representing pathogens', i.e. heat, cold, dryness, wind and damp.

The pulsographs are labelled according to the traditional pulse positions. The following abbreviations are used:

LI	Large Intestine
St	Stomach
TW	Triple Warmer
SI	Small Intestine
GB	Gall Bladder
BL	Bladder
Lu	Lung
Sp	Spleen
Pc	Pericardium
He	Heart
Liv	Liver
Ki	Kidney

Mr R. N.

Complaint: Fourteen year history of dizziness associated with an intense feeling of heat around the neck region.

Commentary

This patient's complaint can be easily understood in terms of traditional Chinese medicine. His predominant pathogen is heat and this is present in all meridians except the gall bladder. Notice the rounded peaks to the deflections, and also note how the recordings of the meridians most severely affected by heat, that is the heart and small intestine, look almost out of control. The gall bladder does show evidence of the pathogen cold due to the predominantly negative deflections; this is an example of two pathogens co-existing with each other, i.e. heat and cold, with heat being dominant. The treatment is to disperse the pathogen heat by using the mother/son law, and therefore to use the earth points on all the meridian pairs affected. This is a serious involvement of the pathogen heat as all the yin (deep) meridians are affected. The points chosen were the earth points on the heart, lung and pericardium meridians (these being the three most seriously affected organs); He7; Lu9 and Pc7.

Mr R. N.
Complaint: Fourteen year history of dizziness associated with
an intense feeling of heat around the neck region.

Left Superficial

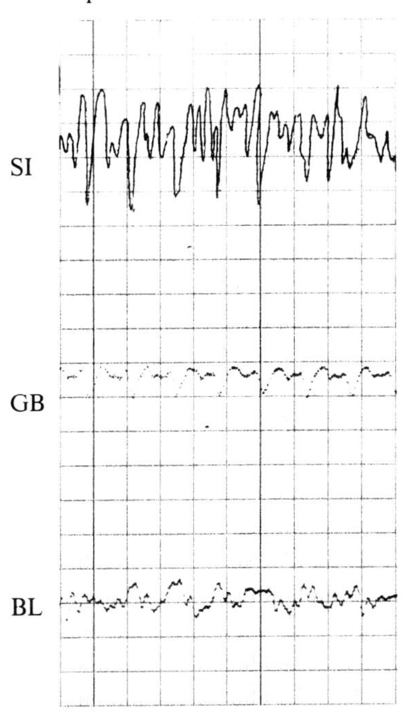

Right Superficial

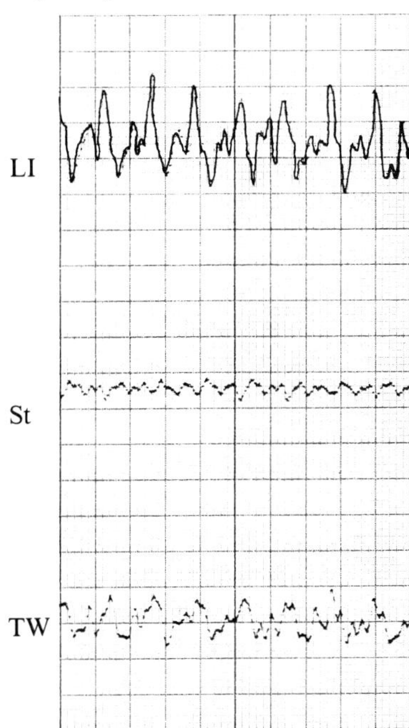

Left Deep

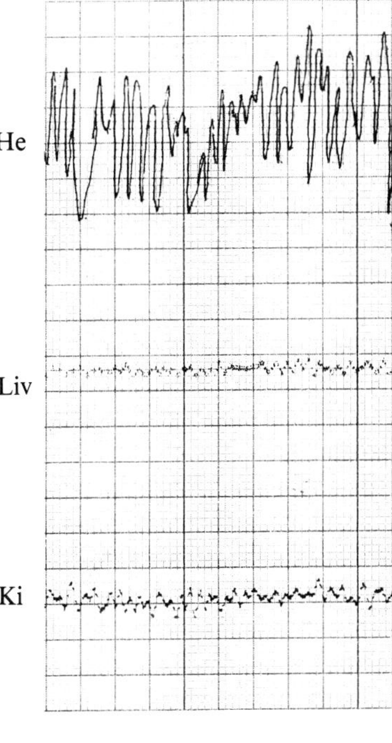

Right Deep

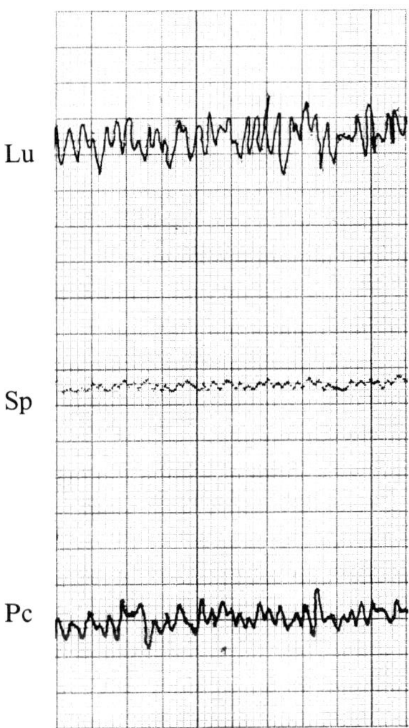

Mrs A. B.

Complaint: Cervical Spondylosis. Also low back pain associated with pain in both hip joints. An X-ray of the lumbo-sacral spine and both hips revealed osteoarthritis present in the lumbo-sacral spine and both hips. This patient also had a duodenal ulcer due to long term analgesic consumption for chronic pain.

Commentary

This pulsograph shows the pathogen cold affecting all the meridians which run over the site of the patient's pain; that is the small intestine and triple warmer meridians for the cervical spondylosis, and the gall bladder and bladder meridians respectively for the hip pain and low back pain.

The patient also has the pathogen heat affecting the spleen and liver meridians and to a lesser extent the stomach meridian. The pericardium meridian also shows some evidence of the pathogen heat. Note on the spleen meridian rounded waves between pulse complexes, this indicates inflammation. These rounded waves are also present on the liver meridian, and to a slight extent on the stomach meridian. This is in keeping with a diagnosis of duodenal ulcer.

The treatment consisted of Moxa to the back shu points on the gall bladder (Danshu, Urinary Bladder 19), the triple warmer, sometimes called the Sanjiao (Sanjiao Shu, Urinary Bladder 22), the small intestine (Xiao Chang Shu, Urinary Bladder 27), and the urinary bladder (Pang guang Shu, Urinary Bladder 28).

Heat must be dispersed from the spleen and liver meridians therefore the earth point according to the law of the five elements must be used on each of these two meridians, so the two points to use in this case are Sp3 and Li3.

Moxa would also be used on a local tender point basis, as this would be standard practice in traditional Chinese medicine if the pathogen cold is affecting any local area.

Mrs A. B.
Complaint: Cervical spondylosis.

Left Superficial

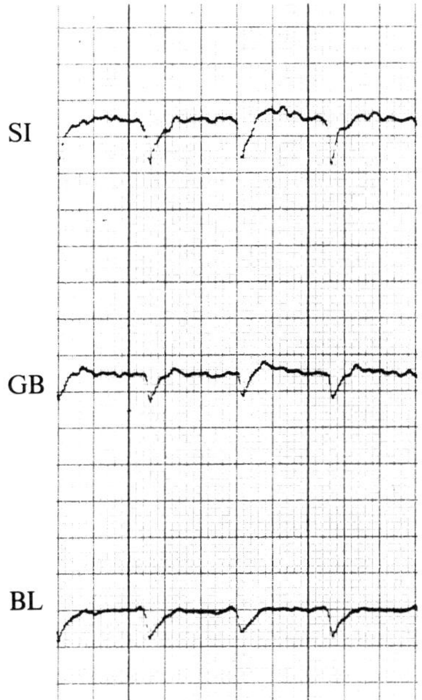

Right Superficial

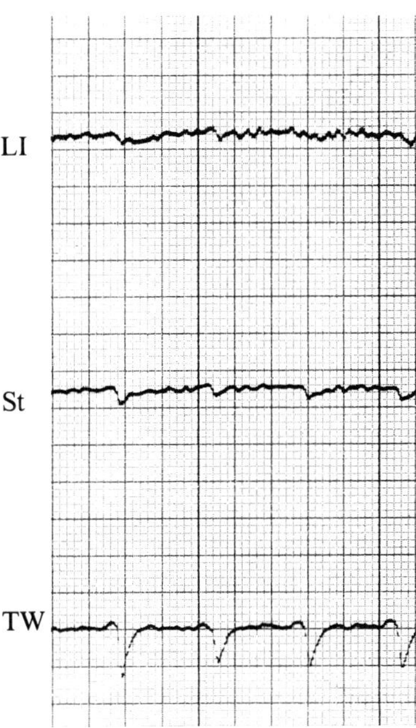

Left Deep

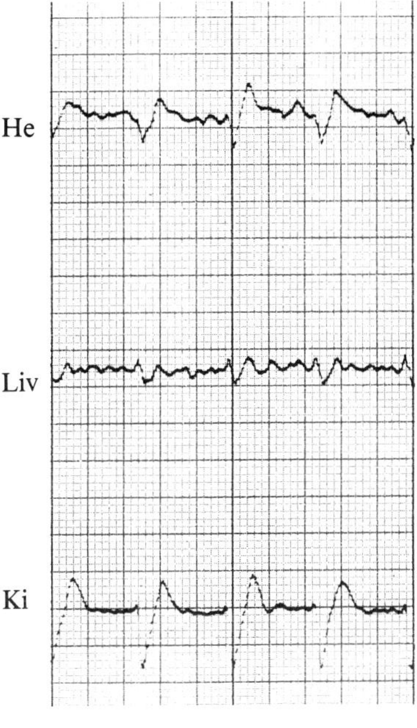

Right Deep

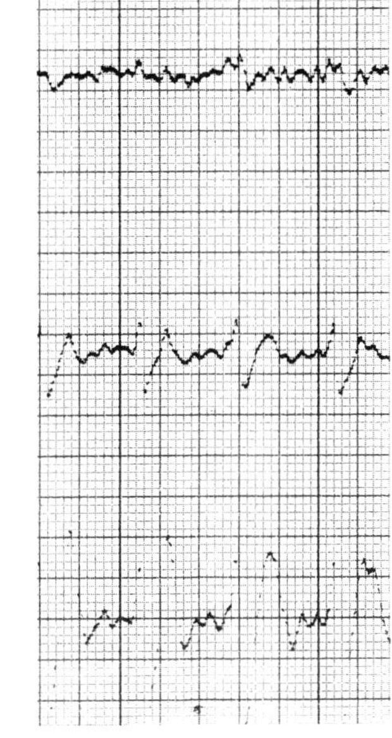

Mr E. T.

Complaint: Raynaud's Syndrome.

Commentary

The major pathogen here is cold as all the deflections are in a negative (yin) direction. Also, there is evidence of energy accumulation in the pericardium meridian. Note the widened complex with a predominantly negative direction in the pericardium meridian with almost two peaks on each pulse complex on the negative wave. This is in keeping with a diagnosis of Raynaud's phenomena, which primarily affects the blood vessels, and which is worsened by cold. Cold is affecting all meridians. Therefore, the treatment is to use moxa on the back shu point on the most badly affected meridians which are the liver, spleen and pericardium meridians. Using moxa for these points will take care of the cold affecting their paired superficial meridian, i.e. gall bladder for the liver; stomach for the spleen, and the triple warmer for the pericardium. Also the energy accumulation ought to be dispersed in the pericardium meridian by using its sedation point Pc7.

Mr E. T.
Complaint: Raynaud's syndrome.

Left Superficial

Right Superficial

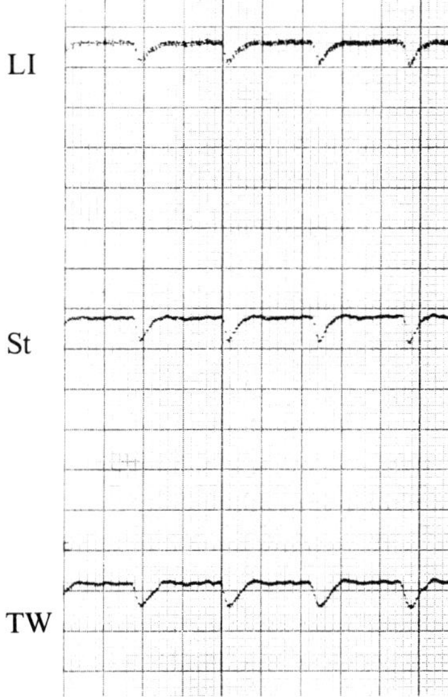

Left Deep

Right Deep

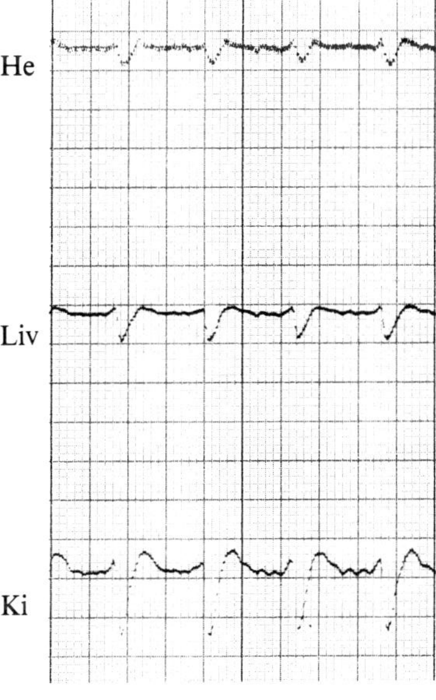

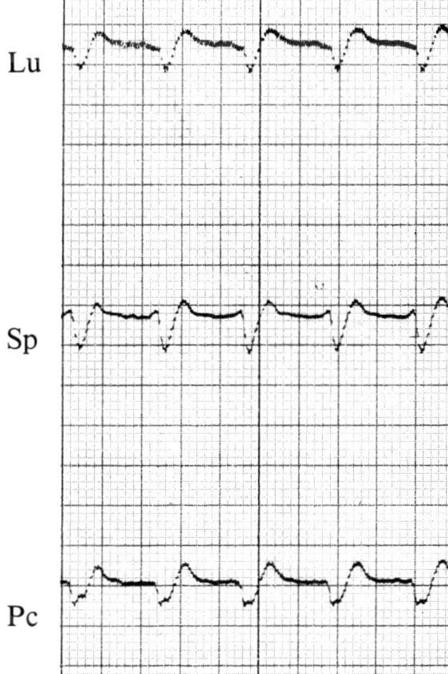

Mrs D. T.

Complaint: Anxiety neurosis leading to nervous breakdown.

Commentary
This pulsograph shows the pathogen wind affecting the stomach, spleen, pericardium, gall bladder, liver and kidney. The pulse shape shown is a typical tense pulse and is regularly seen in patients who have anxiety.

Wind belongs to the evolutive phase wood. Therefore, according to the mother/son law, the fire points on each of the affected meridians should be used. In this case it was decided to choose the yin meridians of each affected meridian pair (paired in the sense of deep/superficial on the pulse measurement points). This is rationalized by the fact that wind is a yang pathogen, therefore, the points used were Sp2, Pc8, Li2 and Ki2.

Mrs D. T.

Complaint: Anxiety neurosis leading to nervous breakdown.

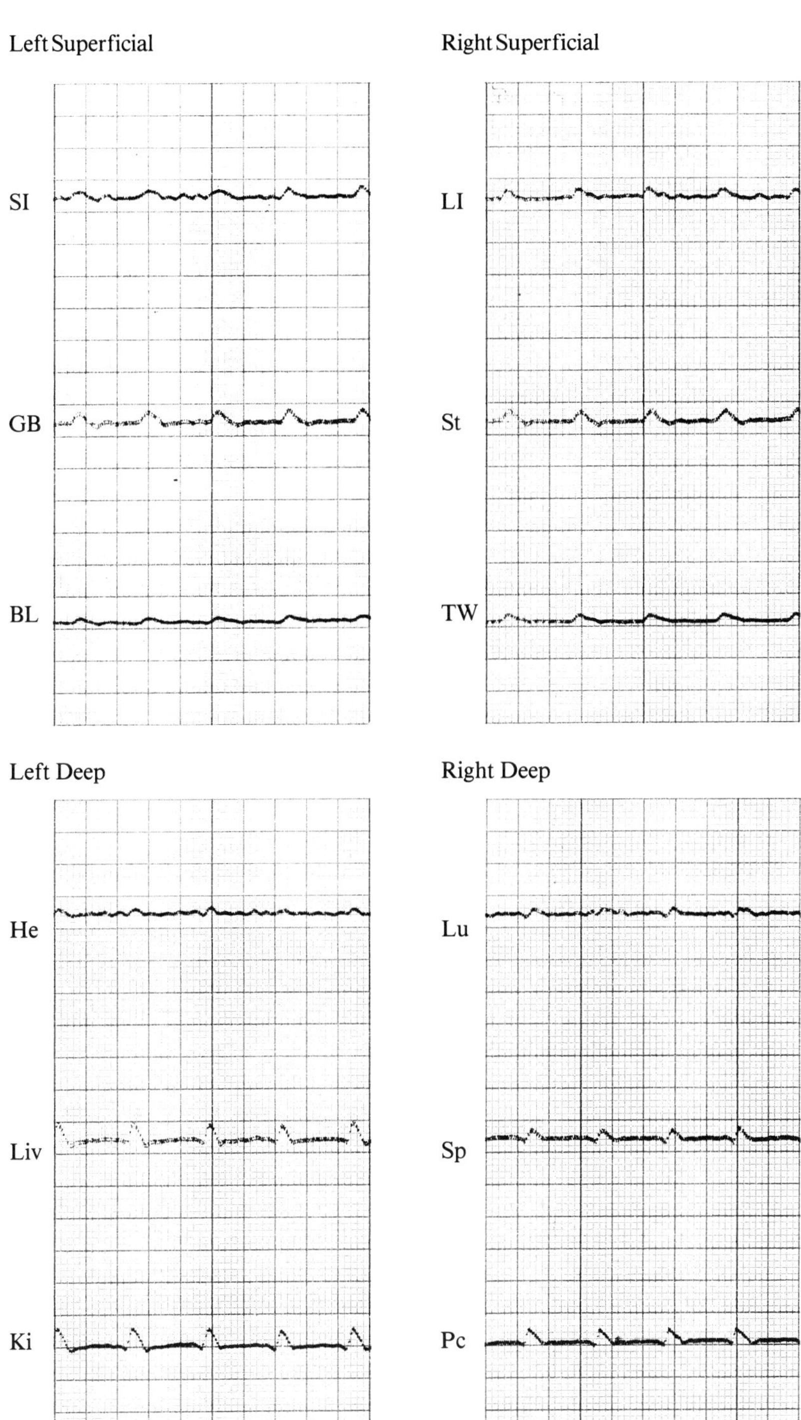

Mr V. H.

Complaint: Hypertension.

Commentary

This pulsograph shows aggressive energy present in the liver meridian, which is violating the lung. As can be seen the lung meridian has a relatively large pulse complex. Also this aggressive energy may overcheck (via the K'o or checking cycle) the evolutive phase earth which is beginning to show this effect, as the stomach meridian here is low in energy. A less important problem on this pulsograph is that the kidney and bladder meridians are empty of energy.

The most important abnormality to correct is to disperse the aggressive energy in the liver meridian by using the sedative point (Li2). Earth also has to be tonified, and this ought to be done using a yin meridian, therefore Sp2 (tonification point of the spleen meridian) was used. Via the mother/son law Sp2 will strengthen the lungs (metal) also, and clearly this is useful as aggressive liver energy is violating the lungs.

Lastly the kidney and bladder ought to be tonified by the yin meridian of this pair (kidney). Therefore, the tonification point on the kidney meridian (Ki7) is used.

Mr V. H.
Complaint: Hypertension.

Left Superficial

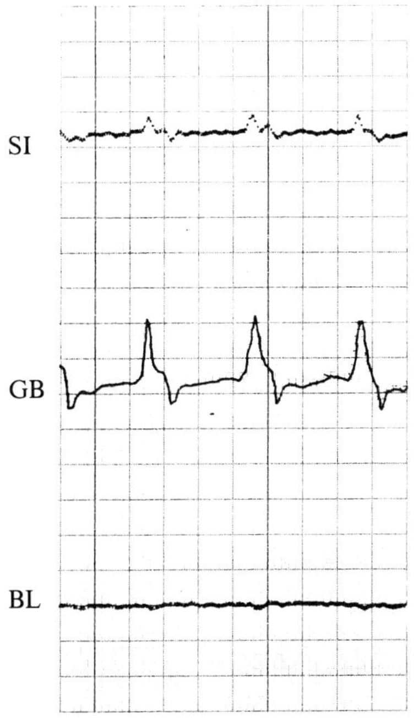

Right Superficial

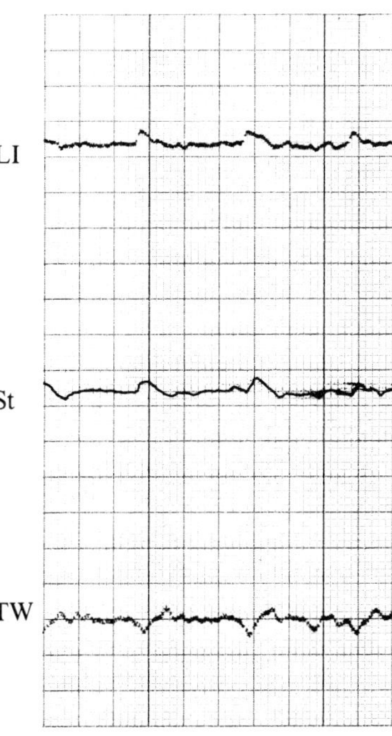

Left Deep

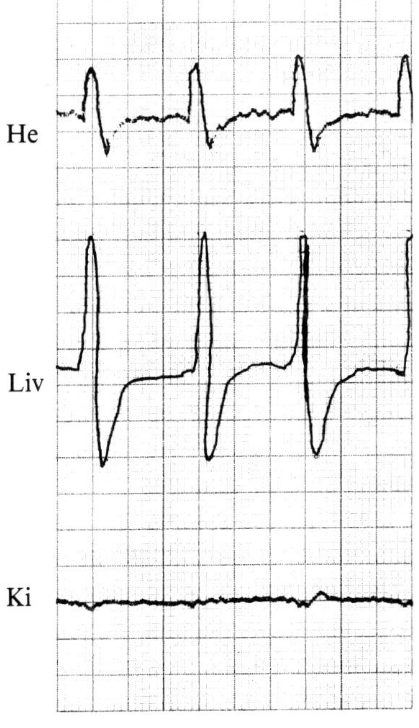

Right Deep

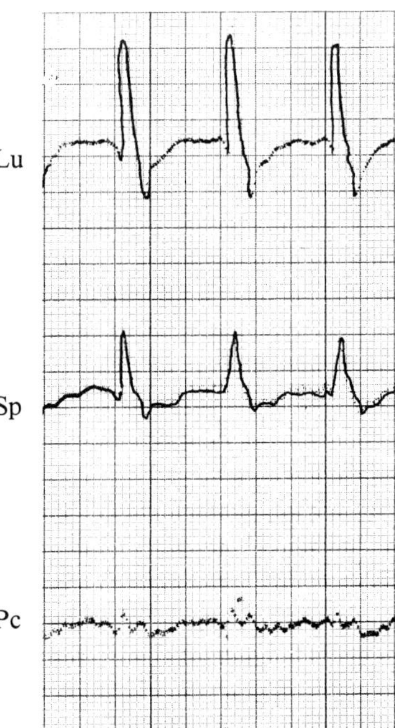

Mr J. D.

Complaint: Vertigo.

Commentary

This pulsograph is another illustration of aggressive energy; in this case aggressive energy is present throughout nearly all the meridians, but it is possible to trace it back to its origins by going through the cycle of the five evolutive phases using the reversed K'o cycle (the violation sequence). On doing this the aggressive energy comes from the kidney and bladder meridians in this case. This has in turn violated the spleen and stomach (earth) which has in turn violated the liver and gall bladder (wood) which has violated the lung and large intestine (metal), and only at this point can we see definite peaks that are only present in the positive deflections on the lung meridian. All the other meridians show a horizontal line at the top of each peak, both in a positive and negative direction. This horizontal line is an artefact arising because the recording pen has reached the limit of its travel. On the continuous readout, using the oscilloscope unit, the deflexions were largest on the kidney and bladder meridians and were slightly less on the spleen and stomach, and less again on the liver and gall bladder. On the paper recording due to the recording pen having limited travel and therefore producing this artefact of the positive and negative peak on this recording, it is only when the aggressive energy has passed through three evolutive phases (earth, wood then metal) that on the third evolutive phase of metal, on the yin (deep position) metal meridian, that is the lung, a positive peak appears which has just come within the limit of travel of the recording pen, yet the negative peak remains beyond the limit of travel.

Aggressive energy has extended from the evolutive phase water, almost through to the final evolutive phase in this sequence, of fire, represented here, on the deep position, by the heart meridian showing a peak present on the positive and negative deflections, indicating that the aggressive energy is beginning to affect the evolutive phase fire at its deep (yin) level. The treatment in this case is to sedate the evolutive phase water at its yin level; that is the kidney. The point used was Ki1. Then all the other evolutive phases should be tonified by the mother/son law. For the earth meridian, Sp2 was used. For the wood phase, Li8 was used. For the metal phase, its yang component (that is the large intestine) was tonified. Therefore, LI11 was used. This was chosen because the aggressive energy on the metal phase had not yet reached the yin level, that is the lung meridian, but had only penetrated to the yang part of the metal phase. The same applied to the fire evolutive phase in which aggressive energy had only penetrated into its yang level; that is the small intestine, therefore the small intestine and not the heart was tonified in the fire evolutive phase. Therefore, SI3 was the last point used.

The above example is a commonly encountered situation of aggressive energy spreading through all the meridians, and this illustrates how the energy must be traced to its source, and its source sedated, whereas all the other phases invaded by the aggressive energy should be tonified to strengthen against attack from aggressive energy. If this is not done the likely interpretation of this pulsograph taken at a superficial level would indicate that all the meridians in which energy excess was present, need sedating. As explained above in the commentary this is not the correct treatment; only the origin of the aggressive energy needs sedating, whereas all the other phases need tonifying.

Mr J. D.
Complaint: Vertigo.

Left Superficial

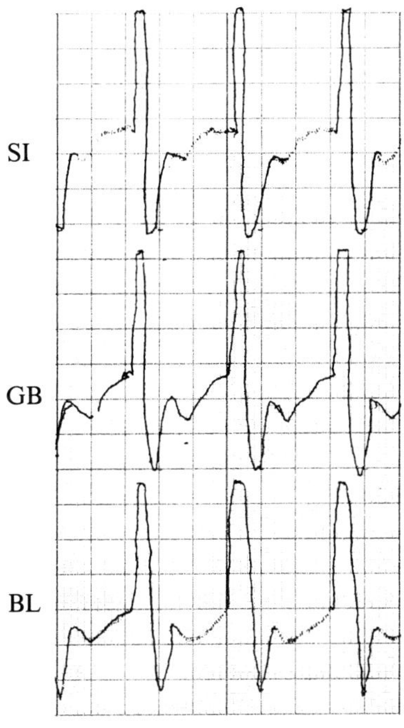

Right Superficial

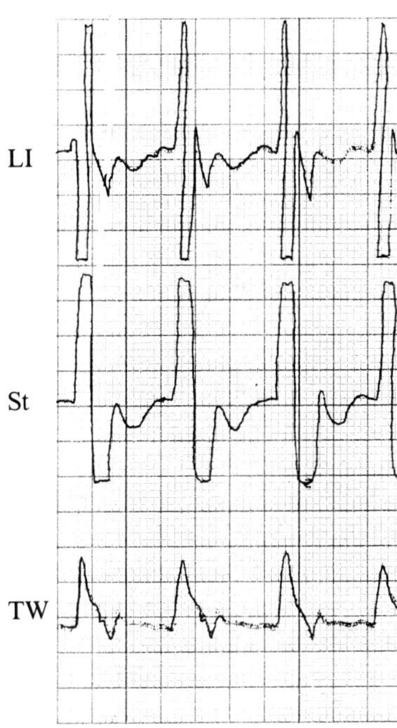

Left Deep

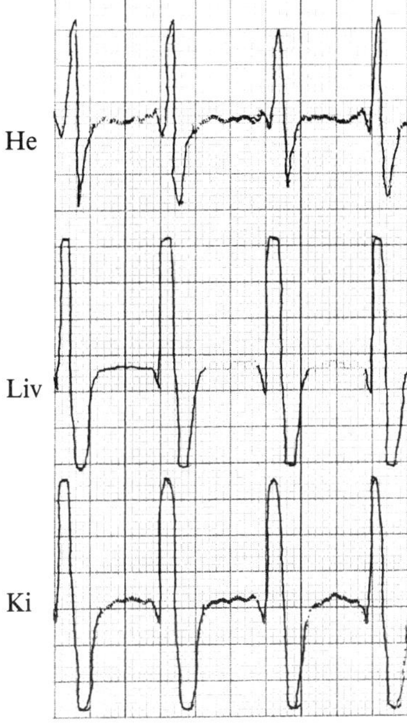

Right Deep

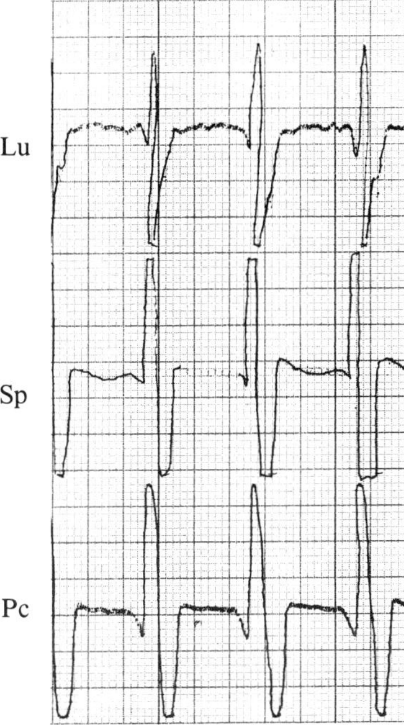

Mr D. S.

Complaint: Eczema.

Commentary

This EPG shows heat in the triple warmer and large intestine meridians. Note particularly the deflections with curved peaks after the main pulse complex in both the triple warmer and large intestine meridians. Also wind is shown affecting the lung, bladder, kidney, heart and small intestine meridians. Heat belongs to the evolutive phase fire, therefore the earth point according to the mother/son law can be used in the triple warmer and large intestine meridians. This leads to a choice of points TW10 and LI11. Wind belongs to the evolutive phase wood therefore the fire points on the affected meridians or in this case, yin meridian of each meridian pair involved can be used. This leads to a choice of the fire points on the lung, kidney and heart meridians. These points are Lu10, Ki2 and He8.

Heat often shows a more florid recording than is shown in the present pulsograph, with many more pre and post waves before and after the main pulse complex.

This EPG also shows some evidence of cold affecting the liver, spleen, and stomach, but this is not the main abnormality and the use of the above points produced a satisfactory result.

Mr D. S.
Complaint: Eczema.

Left Superficial

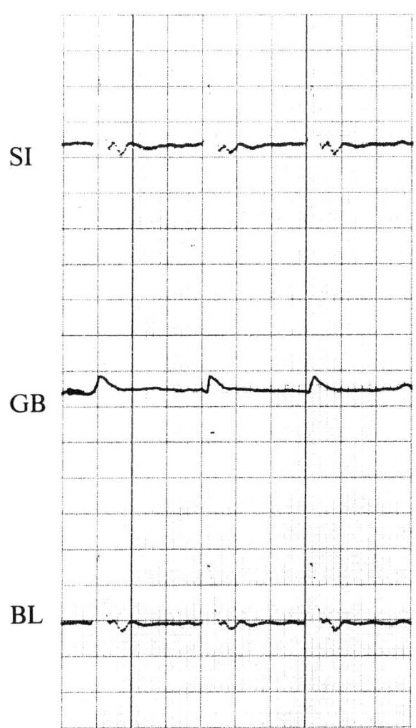

Right Superficial

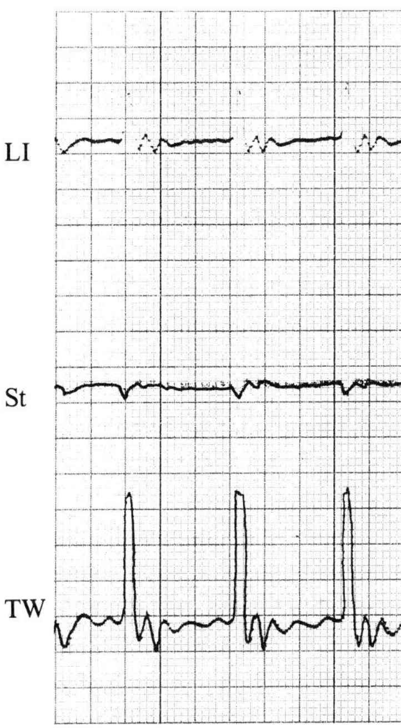

Left Deep

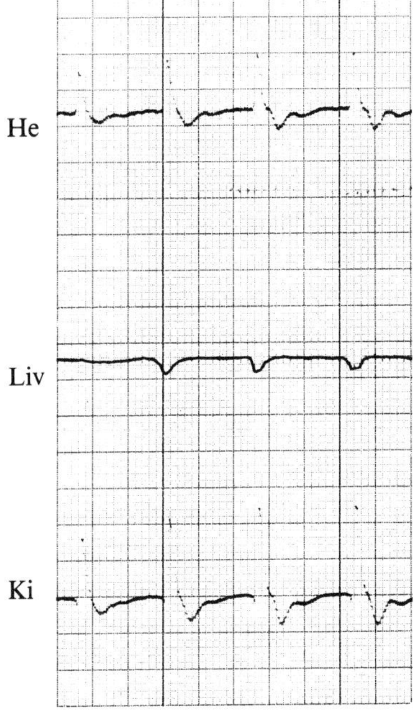

Right Deep

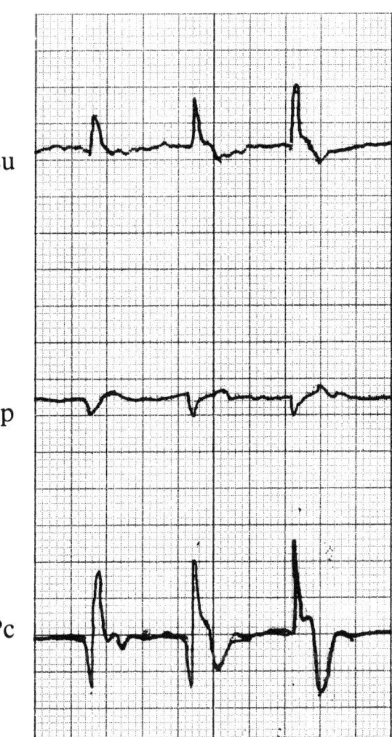

Mrs E. P.

Complaint: Migraine.

Commentary

This pulsograph shows the pathogen wind affecting the small intestine, pericardium, triple warmer, gall bladder and bladder meridians, and also emptiness of energy in the stomach and spleen meridians. Treatment was first attempted using the K'o cycle, so the metal points were chosen on the small intestine, pericardium, triple warmer, gall bladder and bladder meridians, leading to a choice of points of SI1; Pc5; TW1; GB44 and BL67. The spleen meridian was also tonified using point Sp2. This produced no clinical result, just as classical acupuncture based on traditional Chinese diagnosis had not produced any result. On the next appointment it was decided to try using a different law of the five evolutive phases; this time the mother/son law. Therefore the fire points were used on the meridians affected by the pathogen wind, which lead to a choice of points of SI5; Pc8; TW6, GB38 and BL60. The spleen was again tonified using Sp2. This produced a good clinical result within two days of treatment. This patient was having migraines three times a week, but remained symptom free after the second treatment.

The last clinical example provides a particularly striking case of one set of points based on one law producing no effect, whereas a set of points based on a different law did produce a clinical result. In general the author prefers to use the mother/son law as the clinical impression is that it is more effective. Obtaining needling sensation (deqi) is as important with this form of acupuncture as with any other sort of acupuncture involving needling. Electronic pulsography is to be regarded as a particularization of the zang fu abnormality in any given clinical condition, and it enables a more rational and accurate choice of points, and therefore, in the author's view, takes classical acupuncture to the limit of its possible effectiveness.

If no results are obtained following sensible point selection using the EPG, then the author's practice is to try another form of therapy altogether, generally something not related to acupuncture.

If the EPG is to be used with a problem of chronic pain, then local and distant points still have to be chosen in accordance with traditional Chinese teaching, as well as using the points indicated by the pulsograph.

When seeing a patient for the first time, the author's practice is that if, in the first place, acupuncture is considered a suitable therapy for the patient's problem, then a clinical traditional Chinese diagnosis is made, and treatment is based on a point selection using this diagnosis. If no result is obtained then an EPG is recorded; this takes approximately five minutes in experienced hands. Then a more specific point selection is made based upon the EPG, and if pain is the major presenting problem local and distant points are used exactly as they are when a clinical traditional Chinese diagnosis is made. If the patient does not improve after trying at least two possible selections of points based upon the EPG then acupuncture is given up as a mode of therapy.

If the patient does start to improve after application of the points as selected via the EPG, and this is often the case, then no further change of points is necessary. However, on a number of occasions the patient who has been improving using points as selected according to the EPG stops improving; in this case a further EPG must

Mrs E. P.
Complaint: Migraine.

Left Superficial

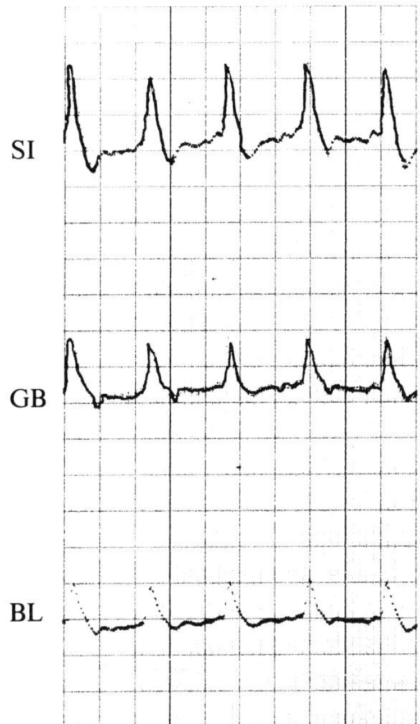

Right Superficial

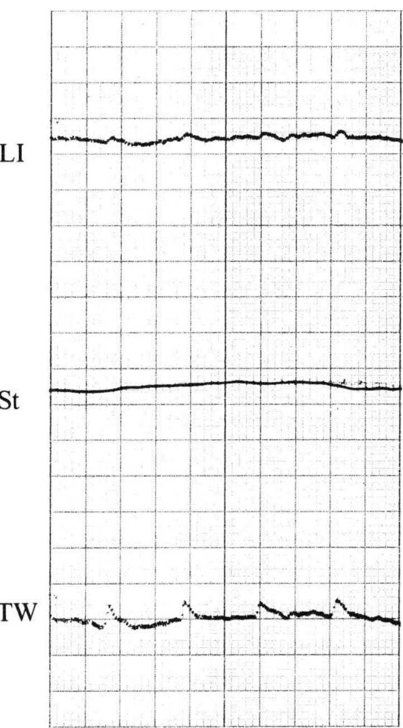

Left Deep

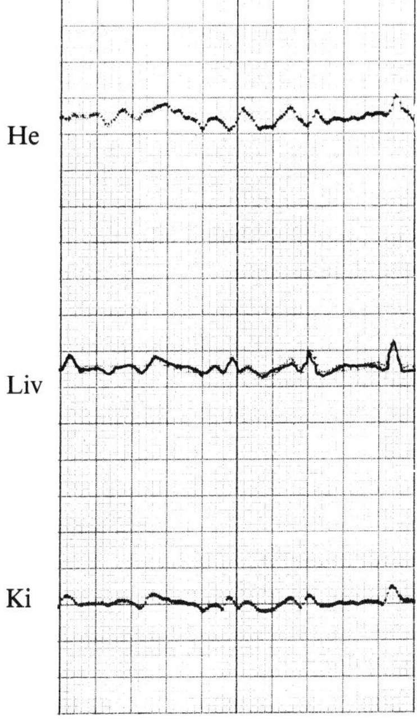

Right Deep

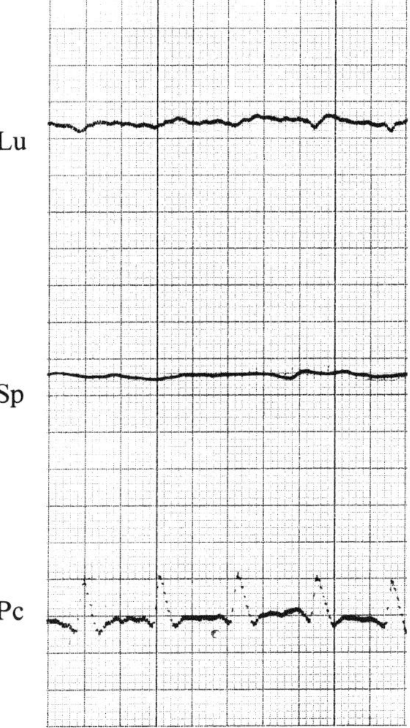

be done and invariably a new situation is seen, in which case a new set of points must be worked out based upon the new EPG, and therapy should continue with the new set of points.

Conclusion Electronic pulsography enables what has been, up to now, a purely traditional Chinese observation to be recorded reproducibly, and this allows a unique opportunity for the investigation in a properly controlled manner of traditional Chinese medical ideas. Such trials would have to be complex, but it should be feasible for them to be designed with every hope that a significant result may be obtained. When designing such trials it should be borne in mind that the possibility remains that the application of the cycles of the five evolutive phases, together with their accompanying laws, may simply be one way of explaining an otherwise inexplicable set of recordings, as without these traditional Chinese explanations the recordings given by the pulsograph would be of no diagnostic or therapeutic use (this represents the null hypothesis). This is not the author's clinical opinion, and evidence against this possibility has been presented in detail here. However, when testing these ideas out in a trial situation the null hypothesis must be regarded as a possibility.

In the author's opinion electronic pulsography, from a practical point of view, carries traditional Chinese medicine to the level of sophistication at which it was originally intended, and indeed, as it probably was applied in ancient China, but sadly, fairly rarely applied by today's acupuncture practitioners, save for a very small number with many years of experience and the privilege of an understanding in depth of the highly complex ideas and theories surrounding traditional Chinese medicine. Pulsography also opens up the possibility that the cycles of the five evolutive phases and their consequent laws may in themselves contain some inherent truth, which as yet has totally eluded both medicine and science.

It is hoped that practitioners who take up pulsography as a result of reading these pages will begin to investigate, in a critical manner, the theoretical foundations of traditional Chinese medicine using the pulsograph as a means of recording these ideas.

Summary A number of clinical examples with EPGs, together with point selection and reasons for such point selection are given. General clinical advice when using electronic pulsography is given. A conclusion to this section suggests that the findings of pulsography could lead to proper investigation of traditional Chinese ideas.

PART TWO

AURICULAR THERAPY
AND AURICULAR MEDICINE

CHAPTER FIVE

AURICULAR THERAPY

Auricular therapy and auricular medicine embody the school of sophisticated ear acupuncture developed by Dr Paul Nogier of Lyon, France, and his colleagues.

Strictly speaking auricular therapy means ear acupuncture without the use of the pulse (see later) and auricular medicine means ear acupuncture with the use of the pulse. In practice the terms are interchangeable. Ear acupuncture has been known to the Chinese for well over 2,000 years, as indeed it has to other ancient cultures, particularly the Egyptians. Dr Paul Nogier, by a number of brilliant discoveries and insights, developed this area of acupuncture into a highly sophisticated system both of diagnosis and therapy.

This section starts with basic concepts, commencing with simple ear acupuncture, as taught by Nogier; then the auricular cardiac reflex is introduced. In the field of acupuncture in particular, and most probably of medicine in general, the auricular cardiac reflex (ACR) represents a fundamentally important and significant physical sign. It is to the everlasting credit of Dr Nogier that his discovery of the ACR should occupy such an important position in auricular medicine, even though as yet its wider significance has been realized by only a very small number of doctors. However, it continues to be a focus of controversy.

Auricular therapy and auricular medicine can be divided into two main schools; the French school headed by Dr Paul Nogier, and the German school influenced largely by Dr Frank Bahr. The main differences between the two schools lies in the use of filters. The French school uses many filters and the teaching tends to be complicated and confused but nevertheless valid in practice, that is if the practitioner is able to remember all the necessary details when approaching any particular clinical situation. The German school has simplified Nogier's teachings and teaches a practice of auricular therapy and auricular medicine based on the use of as few filters as possible. In the author's view this leads to clearer teaching and to better therapeutic application of the method. This section on auricular therapy and auricular medicine reflects this more simple approach.

The French school under Nogier tends to teach five or six different methods of obtaining one piece of diagnostic information; in other words there are many valid ways of detecting disturbances of laterality but it is not necessary to learn all of them, even though each in itself is valid. For the sake of clarity it is more practical to learn one method, and apply this as a routine.

The author has attempted to draw out general principles in so far as this is possible. This has meant leaving out a lot of detail, especially as taught by the French school under Nogier. This particularly applies when speaking of the newest concepts in auricular medicine (see Chapter 21). A vast amount of new information is available, with a tendency to use more and more filters. Unfortunately this information tends to be complicated and confusing, and in some cases contradictory, so only concepts which have direct clinical usefulness are discussed.

CHAPTER SIX

HISTORY OF AURICULAR THERAPY

Dr Paul Nogier, working in Lyon, France, in the early 1950s came across a number of his patients who had been suffering from intractable sciatica, and noticed that they seemed to get better spontaneously. On further investigation he found that an area at the upper end of the anti-helix of the ear, on the side of their sciatica, had been cauterized. He eventually traced these cases to a lay practitioner working in the countryside near to Lyon. His curiosity aroused by this observation, he decided to search the literature, to see whether this practice had been recorded, and indeed found that it had. He noted no less than nineteen specific references to this practice in French medical literature from 1850 to 1860.[1] This practice died out towards the end of the 1870s and was not recorded again in French medical literature. On further searching Nogier found that Hippocrates reported the use of the ear, and implied that it could be useful therapeutically. Further searches of the literature turned up the interesting practice of cauterizing the ear used by the Egyptians more than 2,000 years ago, in which a small grooved piece of metal with a hole drilled through was used. This was placed over the top of the anti-helix, the hole overlying the area to be cauterized for the treatment of sciatica, the cautery was then introduced through the hole. This practice is recorded in some Egyptian tomb paintings.

Being sufficiently interested in these findings Nogier decided to search the ears of patients with painful conditions, and noted that acutely tender areas were present on particular parts of the ear, depending on where the pain was situated. Slowly a map of the body (homunculus) was built up on the ear.

This was Nogier's first real insight into ear acupuncture. The detection of tender areas on the ear has been well known to the Chinese for many centuries, but the Chinese somatotopic mapping of the ear fails to show any indication of an organized homunculus being present on the ear. In a typically oriental fashion a complicated somatotopic mapping on the ear is shown on Chinese ear maps, with a failure to draw out any underlying principle. Nogier's discovery of a homunculus on the ear, with the head lowermost on the earlobe and the spine situated on the anti-helix, in one stroke removed any necessity to learn all the many points on the ear which the Chinese say exist, as all that has to be remembered is a picture of an upside down foetus projected onto the ear.

Nogier presented this discovery at the first Congress of the Société Méditerranée d'Acupuncture in February 1956. A report of this meeting was written in German by a Dr Bachman of Munich, and from there, reports of Nogier's work reached China and eventually reached the pages of Chinese textbooks on ear acupuncture.[2]

The name auricular therapy was then given to ear acupuncture, which simply consists of needling tender points on the ear, with gold or silver needles. At that time the reasons for using gold or silver needles were unclear; it was simply noted by Nogier and his small band of followers that in some cases, one metal would produce a better result than the other, and occasionally, in some cases, either gold or silver would make the condition worse.

The discipline of auricular therapy remained relatively static until the discovery of the auricular cardiac reflex by Nogier in 1966. The auricular cardiac reflex is a measure of the response of an integrated biological system, such as the body, to any incoming stimulus. Nogier soon realized its potential in diagnosis, and in determination of therapy. From the late 1960s the discipline of auricular therapy was given the new name of auricular medicine, which at that time was a high-sounding name for a partisan but useful approach to acupuncture.

From the late 1960s auricular medicine progressed by leaps and bounds and has now developed into a systematized core of knowledge covering treatment of disease via the ear, using needles, magnetic fields and lasers. Unfortunately, developments in this field of medicine have proceeded with very little rigorous scientific control and with many people trying to prove new theories rather than being concerned with consolidating the basic core of knowledge. The following chapters in this section on auricular therapy attempt to do this, and thereby stimulate the interest of practitioners to first of all learn the method in depth, and then to investigate in a properly controlled scientific manner the findings of auricular medicine.

CHAPTER SEVEN

SOMATOTOPIC MAPPING OF THE EAR

The body is represented on the ear in an upside-down fashion, with the head being represented by the earlobe; the anti-helix representing the spinal column; and the concha representing endodermal structures, i.e. the viscera. The area between the anti-helix and the helix represents mesodermal structures, i.e. bones and muscles, and the helix itself, including the earlobe representing ectodermal structures, such as the spinal column and brain. The division of these three areas of the ear into the representation of ectodermal, endodermal and mesodermal structures is important, and its value will become clear when discussing the three phases on the auricle (see Chapter 21).

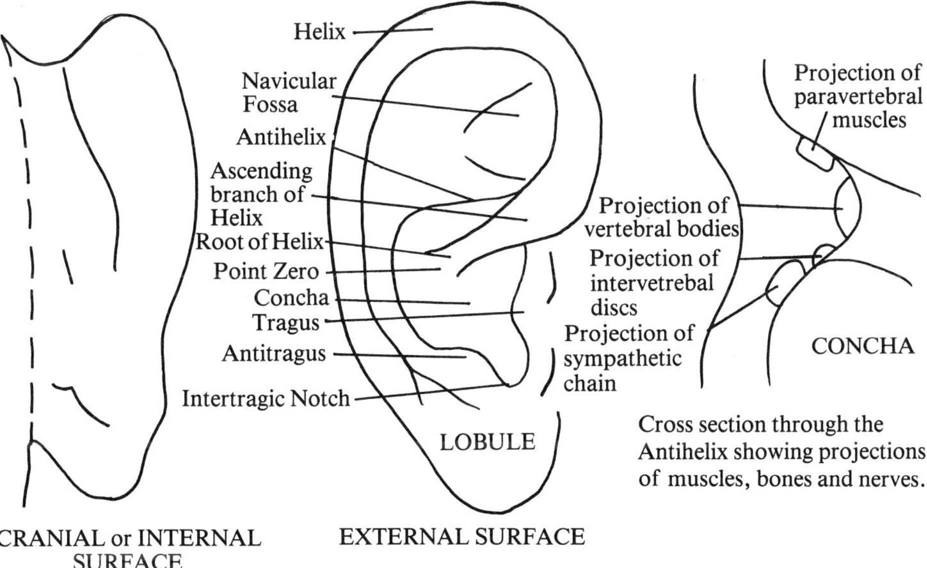

Figure 40. Anatomy of the auricle.

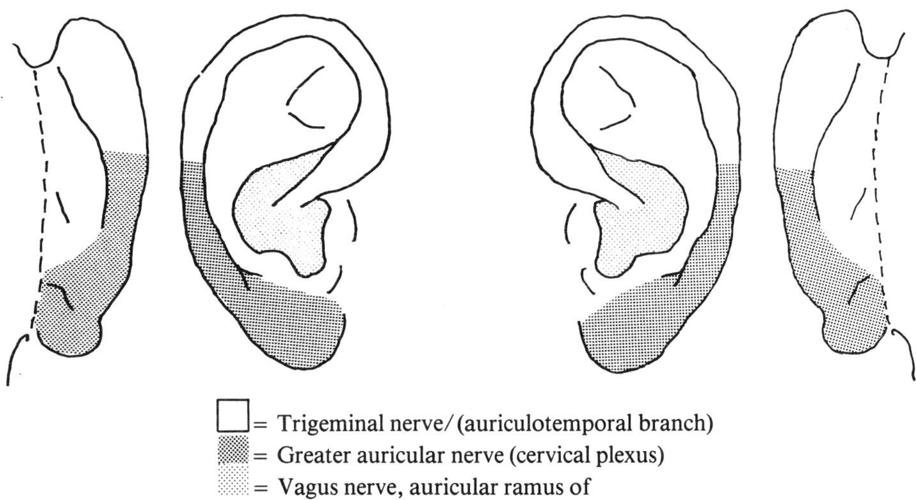

Figure 41.   Nerve supply of the auricle.

The innervation of the auricle is a matter of some debate, but the consensus of opinion is that the concha is supplied by the vagus nerve; the area between the anti-helix and the helix is innervated by the trigeminal nerve, and the remainder is innervated by the superficial cervical plexus (see Figure 41).

The homunculus on the ear is represented in Figure 42. There are several

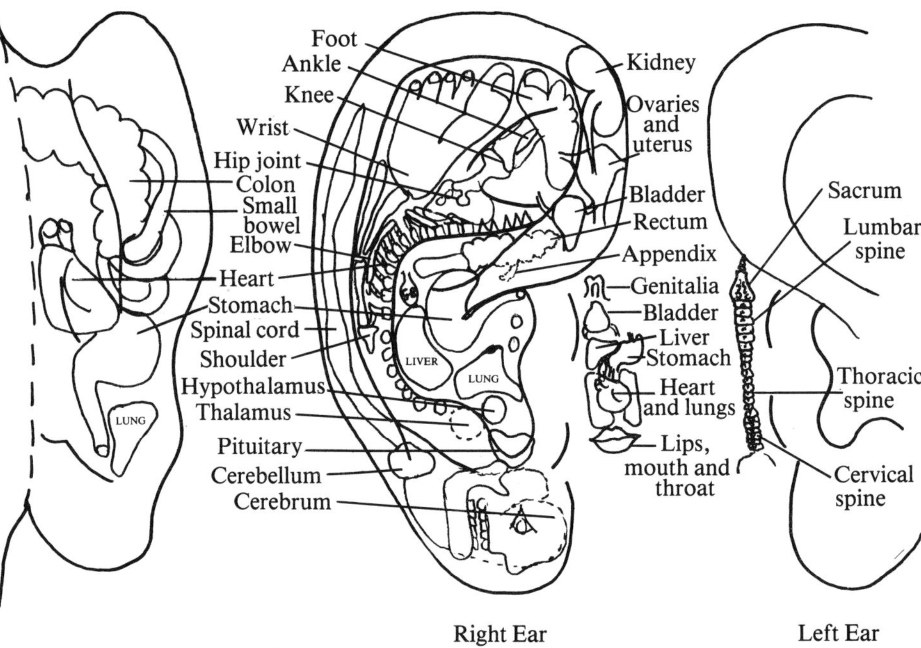

Figure 42.   Ear homunculus in classical upside down position, right-handed subject (after Nogier).

important features to note, the most important of which has been mentioned earlier, i.e. that the head is represented on the earlobe and the spine on the anti-helix. The spinal cord is represented on the helix. The representation of the upper and lower limbs is clear from the diagram. Some textbooks on ear acupuncture go into unnecessary detail into the localization of particular points, with reference to particular areas of the body! As long as the idea of an upside down foetus is remembered, together with the details noted here, then little more is necessary.

Certain points are noted for specific effects but in the author's view auricular therapy tends to take these points to unreasonable lengths such as labelling points as 'worry points', or 'anti-aggression points', or 'sleep points', etc. All that need be remembered is that as the cranium is represented over the earlobe, then it is in this area that points, for example, likely to relieve anxiety or vertigo, or help a patient sleep, are likely to be situated.

The thalamus is projected on the anti-tragus both on the external and the concha surface of the anti-tragus. The pituitary gland is projected on the inter-tragic notch, being predominantly represented on the concha side of this notch. It is clearly in this area that needling may affect endocrine function, and it is the area where the so-called 'gonadotrophic', 'thyroid stimulating hormone', 'adreno cortico trophic hormone', and the 'prolactin' points are situated.

The tragus represents the midline of the body; this area is not given any somatotopic representation on most ear maps which have so far been produced. The right tragus of a right handed individual corresponds with the Renmo (Conception Vessel); that is therefore the anterior midline of the body. This representation, just like the representation of the homunculus, is upside down, with the genital representation being situated superiorly and the representation for the upper end of the Conception Vessel, i.e. the area of the lips, is situated inferiorly (see Figure 42). The left tragus in a right handed individual has the Dumo (Governing Vessel) projected onto it; again with the projection being upside down (see Figure 42). The somatotopy of the tragus, as outlined here, only applies in a well lateralized subject. The concept of laterality and its application to auricular therapy will be discussed in detail in a later chapter.

The viscera are represented in the concha (see Figure 42) and they are represented on the outer surface of the concha, as well as on the cranial surface. This also applies to the representation of the rest of the homunculus in that the cranial surface of the ear is also important. In broad terms the lung occupies most of the inferior half of the concha lying below the root of the helix. The area above the root of the helix is occupied by the pancreas, gall bladder and ileum. The stomach straddles the area at the root of the helix. The point situated right at the root of the helix is termed 'point zero' by Nogier, this is an important reference point. As can be seen from Figure 40 this point is situated in the stomach zone of the concha.

The endocrine glands can be influenced by needling at the appropriate level on the anti-helix corresponding to their spinal level; for example, the adrenal glands can be influenced by needling a point approximately opposite the projection of Lumbar 2 on the anti-helix. Similarly, the thyroid gland can be influenced by needling the area on the anti-helix corresponding to the cervical spine. The projection of the endocrine glands lie more on the concha side than towards the helix side of the anti-helix.

It is useful to visualize the anti-helix in cross section, as illustrated in Figure 40.

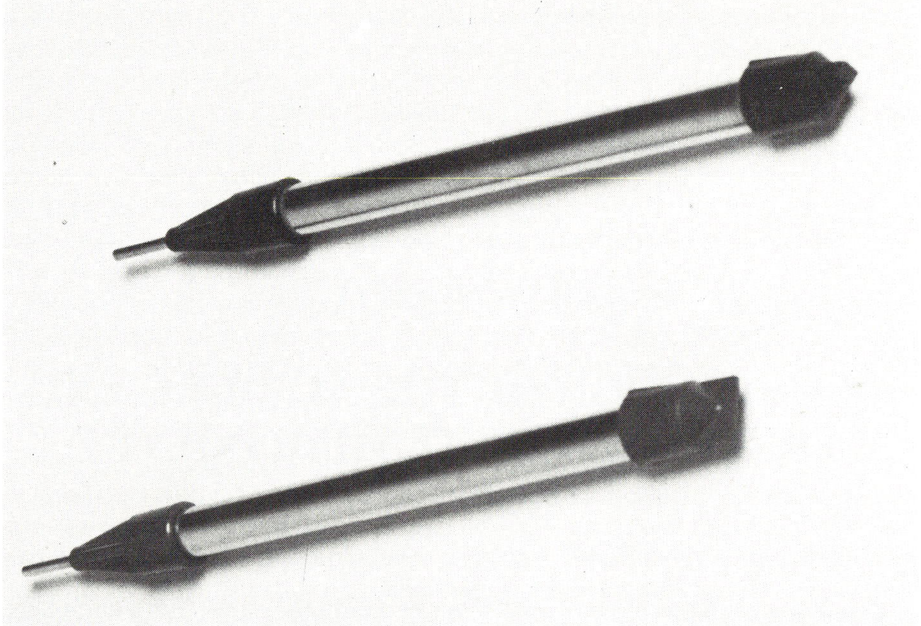

Figure 43.   Pressure palpators: 110 gram above and 250 gram below.

if the pain extends over a wide area, then generally speaking, more than one tender point will be detected. If the tender point detected is not acutely painful then the wrong point has been detected and a further search should be made. Generally speaking, a period of at least a minute is required to detect such a tender point, therefore some patience is required. Those practitioners trying this physical sign out for the first time will soon become impressed with how localized an acutely tender point is when detected on the ear; in other words this is a well defined, clinically useful, and reproducible physical sign.

If no tender point is found on the external surface of the ear, then search on the cranial surface of the ear; this is particularly important as in a number of patients the tender point lies on the cranial surface, and not on the outer surface of the auricle.

Searching the ear with the pressure palpator is illustrated in Figure 44.

Some diagnostic significance regarding the origin of the patient's pain can be made, according to which part of the ear has been found to be tender. For example, in a patient complaining of loin pain, it may be difficult from a clinical point of view to decide as to whether the patient's pain is renal or spinal in origin. Looking at the homunculus on the ear it will be apparent that if the patient's pain is spinal in origin, then tender points should be found round about the area of the second lumbar vertebra on the anti-helix. However, if the patient's pain is renal in origin, then the tender points should be found at the top of the helix. Similarly, if a patient has right-sided abdominal pain, it should be possible to differentiate between a gall bladder problem and an appendicitis, as the tender area for the appendix lies just above the helix, in the depths of the gutter between the helix and the beginning of the anti-helix. Whereas the tender point for the gall bladder lies some distance behind the root of the helix on a level with the upper part of its root.

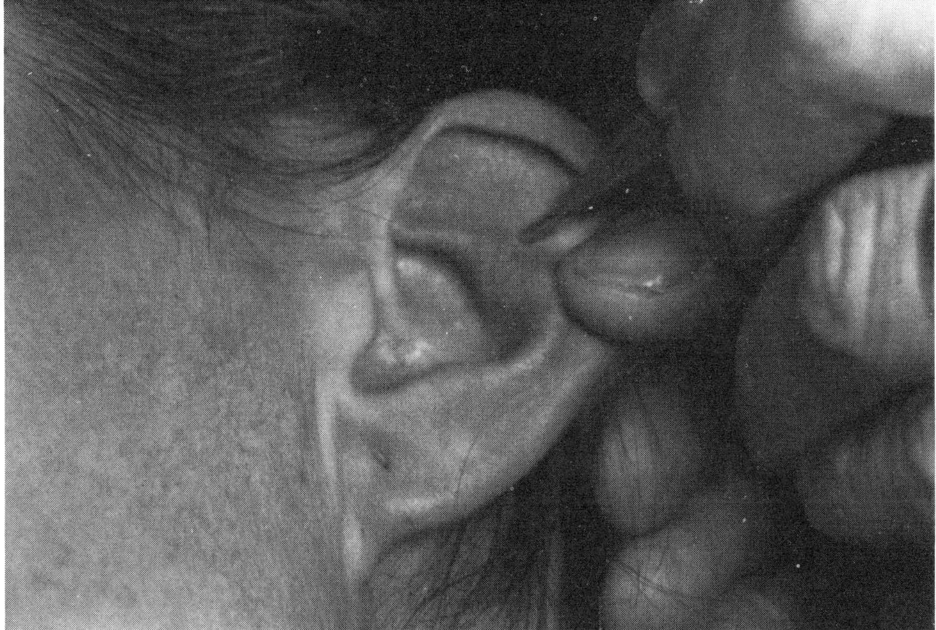

Figure 44.   Searching the ear with the pressure palpator.

There are cases where the situation of a tender point on the ear can be confusing; for example, a patient with a fractured rib will yield a tender point, but it is impossible to differentiate from the area represented by the elbow, as both these sites lie close to each other on the homunculus. Therefore a sensible application of the homunculus should be borne in mind when interpreting sites of tender points on the ear. Many doctors practising auricular therapy claim that often these local ear points are marked by areas of local oedema or perhaps some other change on the skin, such as a local discolouration. In the author's experience this is never a marked phenomenon, and as the clinical sign of the acutely tender point is so easily elicited, then searching the ear using a magnifying glass is generally a waste of time.

Once the acutely tender point has been found this should be marked so it is not lost whilst picking up a needle in order to treat the point. A felt tip pen with as fine a tip as possible is an admirable instrument for this.

Electrical Point Detection on the Ear

For this purpose the *Punctoscope* should be used. This is a simple skin resistance meter with a sensitivity scale, which when turned up to maximum will detect many points, and when turned down to minimum (No. 1 on the sensitivity scale) will detect few, if any, points. For a detailed discussion on skin resistance measurements and their detection the reader is referred to the section on electro-acupuncture in Volume I.

The *Punctoscope* was one of the first point detectors to incorporate the idea of a springloaded measurement probe. This minimizes the possibility of creating an artefact due to the examiner's pressure on the skin, via the measurement probe. The tip of the probe consists of an inner stylet, surrounded by insulation, which

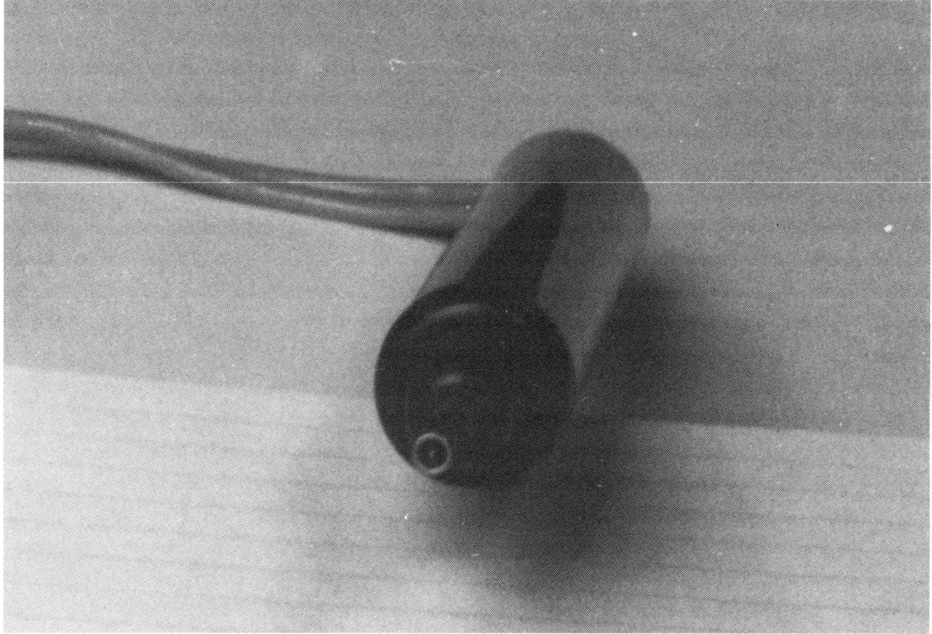

Figure 45.   Tip of *Punctoscope* probe in mode for ear point detection.

separates the stylet from an outer metal cylinder, both of which are springloaded. The outer metal cylinder is retractable using a sleeve which can be slipped over the end of the measurement probe; this then leaves the inner stylet alone projecting. In this mode the *Punctoscope* can be used for body point detection (see Figures 45 and 46).

Whilst detecting ear points the *Punctoscope* is measuring the drop in skin resistance from the outer cylinder to the inner stylet. This resistance drop varies depending on the setting of the sensitivity scale. When sensitivity is set to a maximum, then the skin resistance drop required to work the buzzer will be small whereas if the sensitivity is set to minimum, then the resistance drop will be large in order to produce a detection signal on the instrument. The *Punctoscope* makes a buzzing sound if a point has been detected. If the point has been properly detected a continuous buzz should be emitted from the instrument rather than an intermittent buzzing. The patient should hold the control box of the punctoscope, keeping the springloaded on/off switch towards the handle (i.e. in the 'on' position). This forms one side of the circuit, with the other side of the circuit provided by the measurement probe.

As with searching with the pressure palpator the measurement probe of the *Punctoscope* is carefully and gently pressed in and out over all of the area in which a point is thought to exist. Gentle in and out movement over this area is the best way to find a point. Sliding the measurement tip of the *Punctoscope* around this area will not provide as clear a definition of a point, and is more likely to produce an artefact. Under no circumstances should heavy pressure be used, and no moisture should be introduced onto the ear as this will produce an artefactual lowering of skin resistance. The angle of the tip of the measurement probe to the skin should

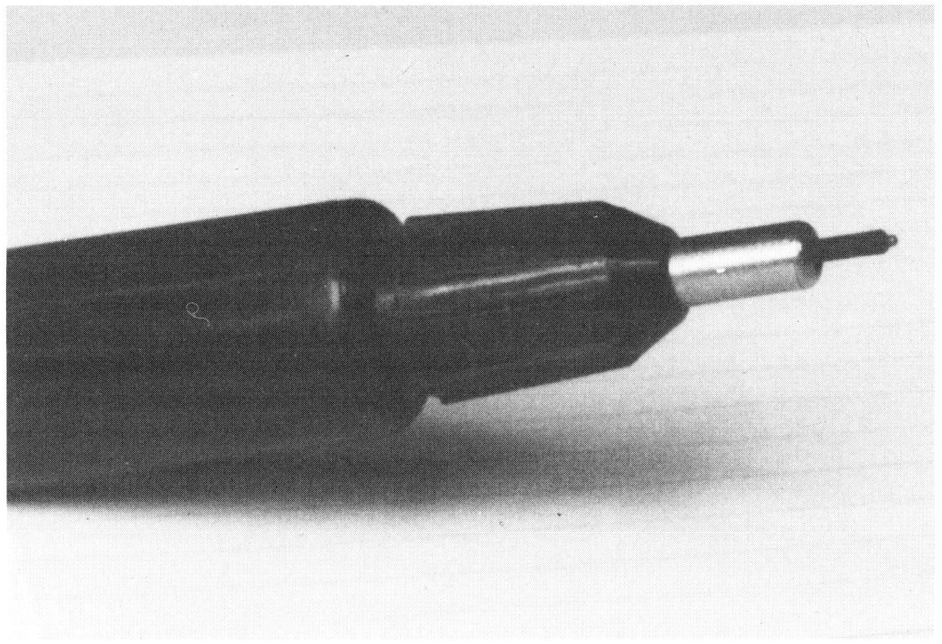

Figure 46.   Tip of *Punctoscope* probe in mode for body point dectector.

be kept as near perpendicular as possible. Angling of the tip of the measurement probe to the skin surface should be avoided.

If no point is found, both on the outer surface and on the cranial surface of the ear, the reason most probably is that the sensitivity on the instrument is too low, and therefore a further search should be made with the sensitivity turned up. Similarly, if many points are detected, then the sensitivity is too high.

Once a point is detected it should be marked with a felt tip pen, just as with point detection using a pressure palpator (see Figure 47).

In painful conditions searching for tender points on the ear with a pressure palpator is the best method as it can be certain that the points so found are the ones that need to be needled, whereas using a *Punctoscope* it is impossible to know if all of the points electrically detected need to be treated, or indeed whether further points exist on the ear which haven't been detected, simply because the sensitivity was too low on the instrument in order to detect these points. However, in non-painful conditions tender points do not necessarily show up on the ear. In these cases electrical point detection, when using ear acupuncture at this elementary level, is a better method of point detection.

The *Punctoscope* also has a facility for detecting points of high skin resistance. In the author's experience these points have no clinical significance.

Treatment of Ear Points

After the ear point has been marked then treatment of this point should be carried out using an inch or a half inch acupuncture needle. The needle should be inserted directly into the point. Generally speaking the practice in Europe is to leave the needle, even in painful conditions, without manipulating it. In Chinese ear

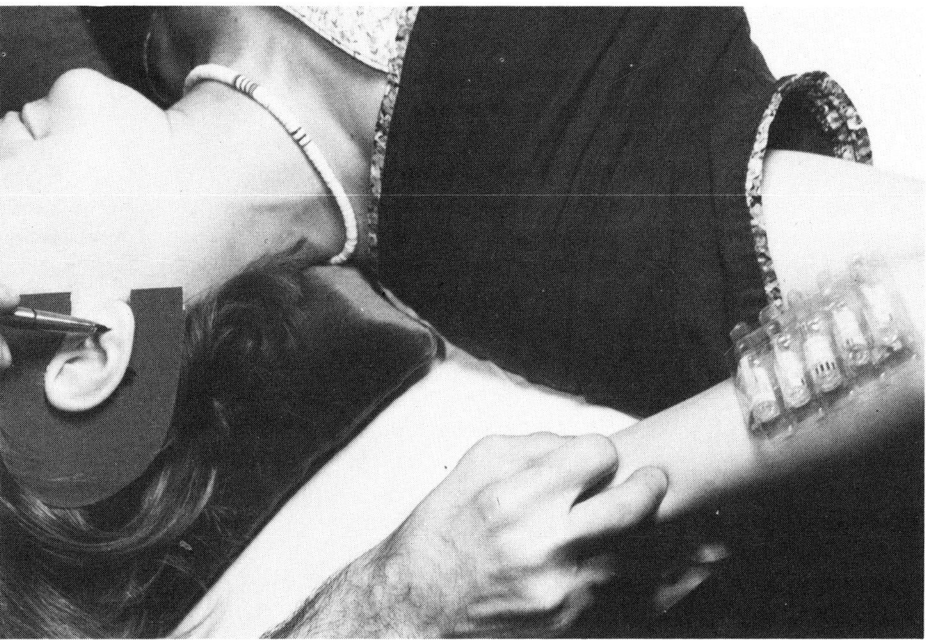

Figure 47. Marking point detected on the ear using a felt tip pen.

acupuncture the needle is gently rotated backwards and forwards when using ear acupuncture for painful conditions. A burning needling sensation is produced, and this sensation is just as important to achieve as when attempting to obtain needling sensation (deqi) when using body acupuncture points. In the author's experience gentle manipulation of the needle in the ear in painful conditions produces better results. For non-painful conditions the needle or needles can be left in place for ten minutes and then removed.

When needling the ear it is important to pay attention to the depth of needling. When a half inch (30 gauge) acupuncture needle is used, and is then left free, it should be inserted far enough so that it will support its length rather than hang. If it does hang when left free it should be gently rotated further into the ear. If an inch needle is used, it should hang slightly. In many cases the tip of a needle will be on the cartilage. There is no case for needling the ear right through from one side to the other. This can be dangerous, and in some circumstances, when the cartilage is pierced, local infection may begin which can be difficult to contain.

The needle or needles should be left in place for approximately ten minutes and then removed, and the patient should be treated at weekly intervals.

Simple ear acupuncture practised at this level is most useful in acutely painful conditions. Some patients with chronic pain, and with non-painful conditions respond better to ear acupuncture than body acupuncture, whereas others don't respond to body acupuncture at all, but respond to ear acupuncture. A common example of this last group of patients, is those who are on steroid therapy for whatever reason. Generally speaking the response to classical acupuncture is attenuated if the patient is on steroids. However, the fact that ear acupuncture works whether the patient is on steroids or not, opens the possibility that ear acupuncture

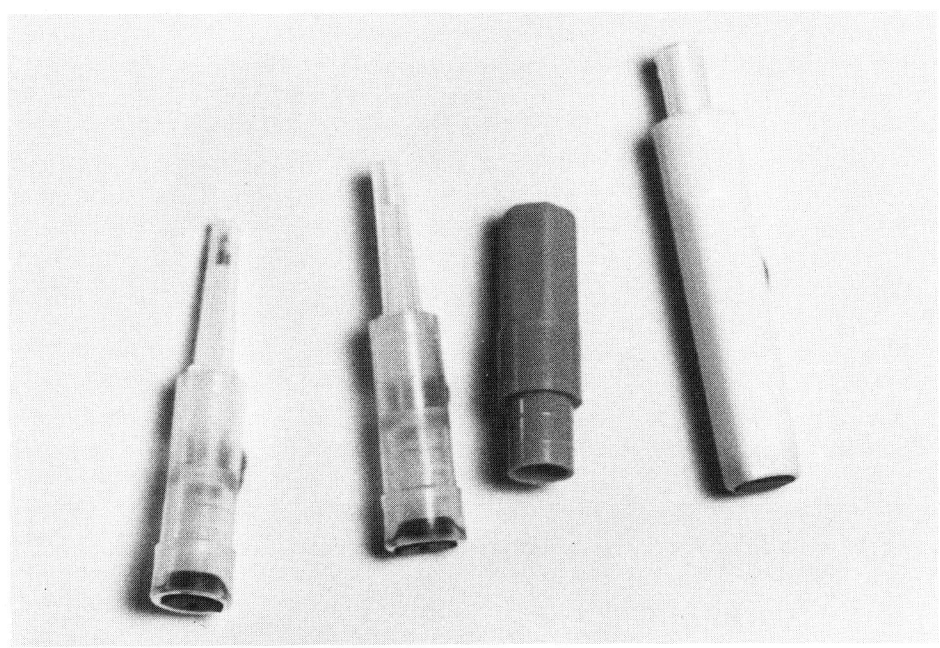

Figure 48.   Semi-permanent needles in their holders. Note: magnet present at the bottom of the holder.

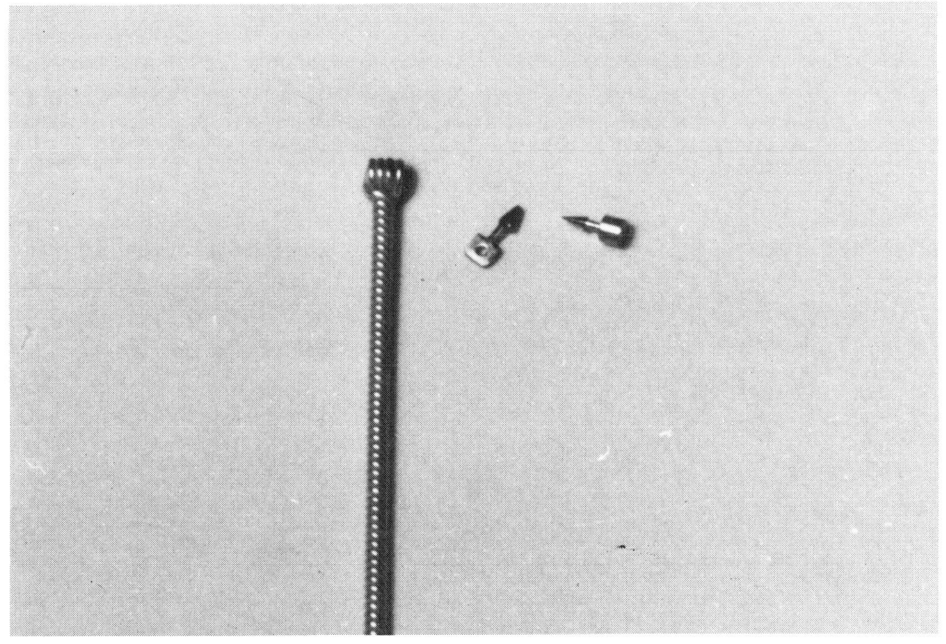

Figure 49.   Semi-permanent needles, one rounded and the other flat, pictured next to the top of an acupuncture needle handle.

is perhaps working through different mechanisms from body acupuncture.

From a practical point of view the advantage of simple ear acupuncture is that it is very quick indeed, pain relief is often immediate, and is as astonishing to the practitioner as it is to the patient. Its disadvantage is that often relief is not as longlasting as when using classical acupuncture, and this can become a problem when using simple ear acupuncture for chronic painful conditions. One way around this problem is to insert a so-called 'semi-permanent' needle into the tender point or points on the ear, and this, in most cases, has the effect of prolonging pain relief. Semi-permanent ear needles are made by Sedatelec, and a photograph of such a needle, next to a handle of a conventional acupuncture needle is shown in Figure 49. As the semi-permanent needle is impossible to handle because it is so small, it is supplied together with an introducer which is simply pressed onto the ear, over the tender spot. The author's practice is to swab the tender spot, and then to put a small amount of antibiotic cream over the point into which the semi-permanent needle will be inserted. Since having followed this practice no problems with infection have arisen in the author's practice, having inserted many thousands of semi-permanent needles. Prior to using antibiotic cream a number of local infections developed following the use of semi-permanent needles. An illustration of the insertion of a semi-permanent needle is shown in Figure 50.

A rapid, firm, and vertically directed thrust is required in order to insert a semi-permanent needle effectively. If the thrust of the needle holder is angled relative to the skin surface, then often the needle only partially penetrates the skin, and either drops out within minutes, or only stays in for a matter of a few days, therefore it is important to hold the needle holder exactly perpendicular to the skin surface, and support the back of the auricle with the free hand.

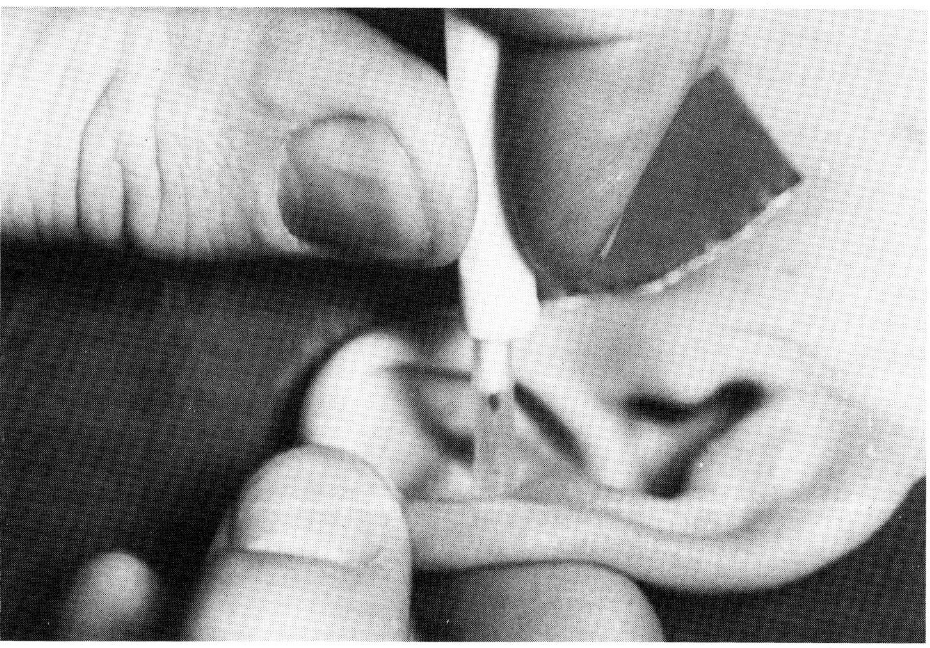

Figure 50.   Insertion of a semi-permanent needle.

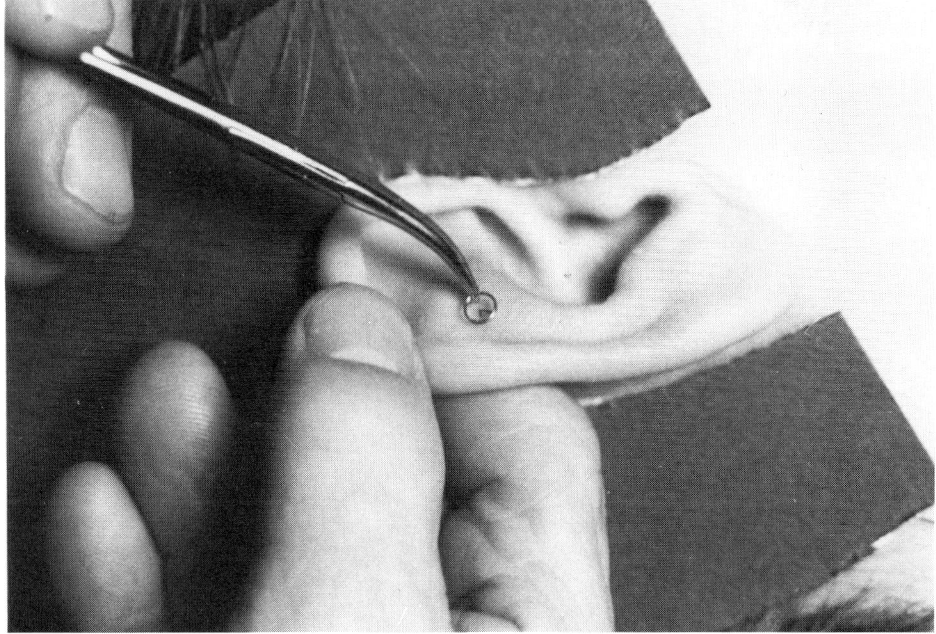

Figure 51.   Insertion of Chinese ear press needle.

Sedatelec's semi-permanent needles remain in on average for 2½ weeks. Their advantage over Chinese earpress needles (illustrated in Figure 51) is that they don't need covering with a plaster to hold them in, whereas earpress needles do. Earpress needles tend to stay in for the same length of time as do Sedat semi-permanent needles, and if large numbers of semi-permanent needles are to be used, then Chinese earpress needles have a cost advantage.

When Chinese earpress needles are used the patient should be instructed to stimulate the needle by placing the thumb behind the area where the needle has been inserted, and the index finger over the top of the needle, and to gently rub it between thumb and index. This should be repeated every time the pain recurs. In a successful placement of such a needle, on stimulation the pain will disappear.

When using a Sedat semi-permanent needle manual stimulation can be used, also magnetic stimulation can be used by the patient using the end of the needle holder in which a small disc magnet is provided (see Figures 48 and 52). This should be rotated over the projecting part of the semi-permanent needle, in a clockwise direction if the needle is inserted in the right ear, and in an anti-clockwise direction if the needle is inserted in the left ear, i.e. the magnet is rotated in a forwards direction, whether the needle is in the right or left ear. This should be done for thirty seconds, three times a day, and also when the patient feels pain.

The use of either semi-permanent needles or Chinese earpress needles can be dramatically effective, and often is so in chronic, intractable painful conditions such as phantom limb pain. It is gratifying to see such good results accruing from a relatively simple procedure. The author, and many colleagues using similar methods have managed a number of previously intractable phantom limb pains using this simple method. Other chronic painful conditions which seem to respond

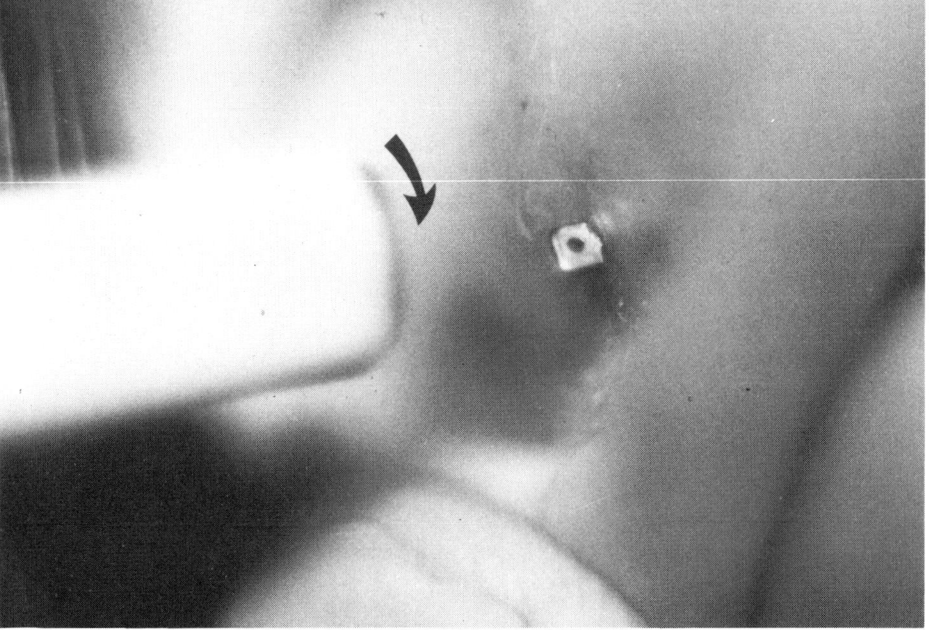

Figure 52. Disc magnet at the end of the needle holder being rotated over a semi-permanent needle. Arrow shows direction of rotation of magnet (for a right ear).

best to semi-permanent needle insertion are painful scars, and chronic pain which has a major autonomic component such as the sympathetic dystrophies.

Two important practical problems arise when using semi-permanent ear needles, and indeed when needling the ear at all. The first is accuracy of needle placement. As all the body is represented on the ear, the points are very close together. Therefore, absolute accuracy in needle placement is of paramount importance. An error of a millimeter may be enough to lose any clinical effect. This is also important when using semi-permanent ear needles. If a patient can only be maintained painfree using semi-permanent ear needles, and there are an appreciable number of intractable pain patients who can only be satisfactorily managed in this manner, then it is clearly not going to be possible to replace the semi-permanent needle in the same point in the ear immediately after the last needle has fallen out. As indicated above the needles generally stay in for approximately 2½ weeks. The most practical solution is to use a mirror image point on the opposite ear. Generally speaking the ear on the side of the pain will work better than the opposite ear. The opposite ear will give some degree of pain relief, if not as great as when using the ear on the same side as the pain. After approximately two weeks the ipsilateral ear to the pain will have recovered enough for reinsertion of a needle.

In some cases, when searching for tender points, or indeed when using the *Punctoscope*, a line of points will be detected, situated on a radius from point zero (this is the point situated where the root of the helix joins the concha). When using semi-permanent needles the point to insert the semi-permanent needle should be the tender point situated farthest out on this radius from point zero. Often, this is situated almost on the edge of the helix. These points tend to produce better relief than points situated more centrally on the radius from point zero.

If no satisfactory relief from pain, or alleviation of the patient's condition if a non-painful condition is being treated, is obtained when using simple ear acupuncture, either using stainless steel needles or semi-permanent ear needles, then ear acupuncture practised at this level will not work, and a more sophisticated approach is necessary. More complex clinical problems can be treated effectively when using the more complicated procedures of auricular medicine, and the remaining chapters in this section will deal with these techniques.

Summary

Point detection using a pressure palpator for finding tender ear points, and also for electrical point detection on the ear are described. The treatment of these points, using stainless steel needles, and semi-permanent ear needles is described.

CHAPTER NINE

AURICULAR MEDICINE: THE AURICULAR CARDIAC REFLEX

The auricular cardiac reflex (ACR) is perhaps the most brilliant and important discovery made by Nogier. It is unclear how the reflex was first discovered but it is apparent that the change in the pulse amplitude was noticed initially on palpating the auricle with the pressure palpator. The name 'auricular cardiac reflex' has no special meaning attached to it, other than the fact that it was first discovered in relation to ear acupuncture. However its usefulness extends far beyond auricular medicine. In recent years different names have been given to the auricular cardiac reflex; perhaps the most common of the new appellations is vascular autonomic system (VAS). In France the auricular therapists call the ACR the RAC (réflexe auriculo-cardiac). Sometimes it is referred to as the 'Nogier reflex'. All these different names serve to confuse, and the original name of auricular cardiac reflex, as described by Nogier in his first book *Treatise of Auricular Therapy* (1972) has been adopted by the author.

In order to understand the ACR it is useful to imagine a pressure wave in an artery which behaves very much like a standing wave. The ACR is easier to understand if it is explained in terms of such a standing wave, and it is a movement in this standing wave, situated in any artery; this movement is generally felt on the radial pulse, but may be felt on any pulse position. It is essentially a manifestation of autonomic change and is in no way to be confused with traditional Chinese pulse diagnosis (see section on Electronic Pulsography).

To further explain the concept of a standing wave in an artery, it is useful to conceive of the artery as being rather like a sausage skin filled with water (see Figure 53). The fixed end of the sausage skin is equivalent to the arteriovenous anastomoses (peripheral resistance), and the opposite end to the proximal end of the artery. During systole the pressure wave is transmitted throughout the arterial system, and therefore into the left-hand end of the sausage skin. The pressure wave is then transmitted along the artery, or in terms of the diagram, through the water within the sausage skin. When the pressure wave reaches the fixed right-hand end (equivalent to peripheral resistance), it is reflected back and therefore a second (reflected) pressure wave is produced. These two waves, travelling in opposite

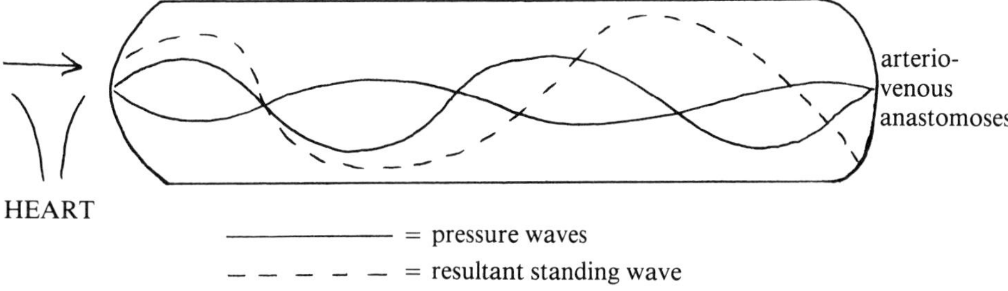

Figure 53.   Conceptualization of an artery as a sausage skin filled with water.

directions, interact with each other, and produce an interference pattern, so that a single resultant wave is formed which has properties similar to a standing wave. A standing wave can be imagined as a wave which neither travels forwards nor backwards, but any particle situated on the standing wave would move in a forwards direction. A standing wave is always the result of an interference pattern. Therefore, in the sausage skin, a series of fixed peaks and troughs is produced.

If the image of the sausage skin full of water is applied to any artery, then a series of standing waves can be visualized as being present in any artery; subject to the variables of heart rate, and the state of the peripheral resistance. Both of these are variable, and are under autonomic control, therefore if the peripheral resistance varies, the positions of the peaks and troughs will move, either proximally or distally. Heart rate seems to make little difference to the movement proximally or distally of the standing wave. Increased heart rates produce more peaks and troughs in any given distance of artery. Therefore, according to this explanation, if any artery was exposed over its whole length, on looking at the artery all of it would appear to be pulsating, whereas if a palpating finger was carefully and slowly run down the artery, at certain points the pulsation would appear to be of greater amplitude than at other points. This can be confirmed on the reader's radial pulse, simply by moving the palpating thumb slowly and gently over the palpable length of the artery, and noticing that at one particular point the radial artery pulse appears maximal, whereas at other points the pulsation is not quite so strong. It is easy to argue that local anatomy surrounding the artery may be responsible for this phenomenon, but when one examines a pulsograph (see section on Electronic Pulsography), it is seen that in some patients, maximal pulsation appears at a position proximal to the radial styloid process (the maximal pulsation is usually thought to occur at the level of the radial styloid process), and in other cases, the point of maximal pulsation is situated distal to the radial styloid process, whilst in another group the point of maximal pulsation lies in the middle position, opposite the radial styloid process. Therefore local anatomy cannot explain why arterial pulsation feels stronger at some points than at others.

A positive ACR is, by convention, taken as meaning a movement distally of the standing wave. It is possible to detect this movement by palpating the pulse. This requires a considerable amount of training in order to be able to perceive a positive, or indeed a negative ACR with as near 100 per cent accuracy as possible. However, the ACR is a physical sign like any other physical sign, which requires a certain amount of skill on the part of the practitioner in order to detect it reliably. In terms

The area of the concha and the 'swimming trunk' area supplied by the sacral parasympathetics falls broadly within such a division. The skin above the clavicle, and indeed on the face and neck becomes more difficult to explain, yet it remains that the ACR produced by shining a light is always opposite to that produced when the light is shone on so-called 'sympathetic skin'. This phenomena has a practical application which is useful when teaching the ACR to doctors who are finding difficulty feeling a positive ACR.

In order to feel an ACR at its maximal it is going to be easiest if a maximal displacement of the standing wave is induced. This can be done by firstly shining the light on sympathetic skin, at which position the standing wave will move distally, and then immediately shining the light on parasympathetic skin, at which position the standing wave will move proximally. There will then be a maximum displacement of the standing wave, and indeed in some cases when the light is shone on parasympathetic skin, after being first shone on sympathetic skin, i.e. from forearm to cheek, then the pulse often appears to disappear altogether for two or three beats after the light has been shone on the parasympathetic skin. These two different ACR reactions are of practical importance when applying the ACR to auricular medicine, and particularly when using the ACR in the diagnosis of allergies (see section on Clinical Ecology).

Determination of Energy Level Using the ACR If a light is shone on an area of skin lying in the so-called sympathetic area, then initially a positive ACR will be felt. If the intensity of the light is increased beyond a certain level, then the ACR becomes negative, and then on decreasing the intensity of light again, the ACR again becomes positive. This is where the rheostat controlled

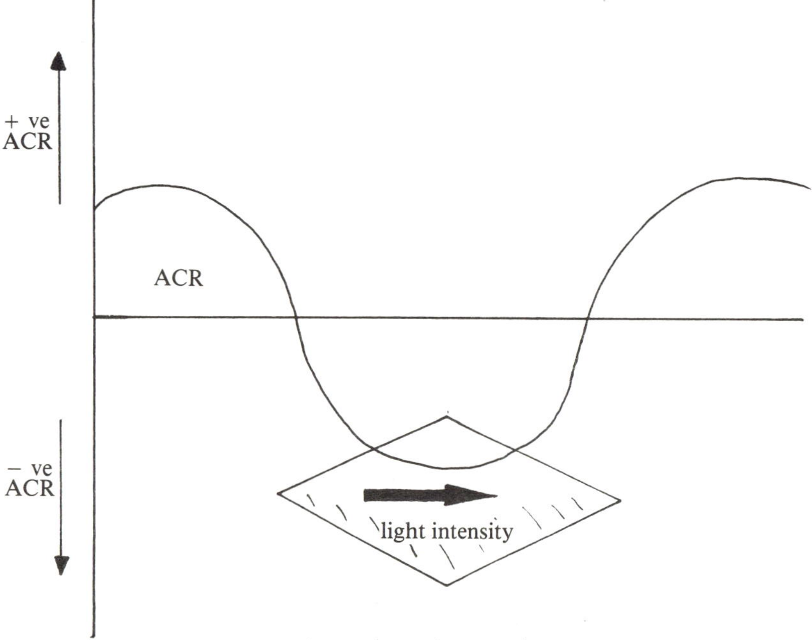

Figure 59. Variation of ACR due to different energy levels applied to the skin.

examining light, such as a Heine light, becomes useful, as by determining which light intensity is employed the energy level of any particular area of skin can be determined (see Figure 59).

During the course of any examination and treatment session the position of the standing wave tends to change slightly, so that the position of the examining thumb may need to be changed from time to time by 'recalibrating' with the Heine light. **Further Observations on the ACR**

From the point of view of comfort of the examiner the author has adapted his examination couches to include a support for the examiner's palpating arm, as in auricular therapy, or indeed when using the ACR in diagnosing allergens the radial pulse needs to be felt for periods in excess of ten minutes. This adaption is illustrated in Figures 59a and 59b.

As the position of the standing wave of the radial pulse is under autonomic control, being independent on how open or closed the arteriovenous anastomoses are, and as the ACR reaction depends on whether the light is shone on sympathetic or parasympathetic skin, a positive ACR is sometimes called a sympathetic ACR, and a negative ACR a parasympathetic ACR. *The ACR can therefore be considered as a measure of autonomic response.*

The ACR is both a qualitative and quantitative response to a stimulus; qualitative in terms of how much the amplitude of the pulse increases or decreases, depending whether a positive or a negative ACR is palpated, and quantitative in respect of the number of pulse beats for which the ACR remains positive. This last physical sign is more difficult to detect, as it is often not obvious when the ACR goes from positive back to a normal pulse again. The author would dissuade practitioners from

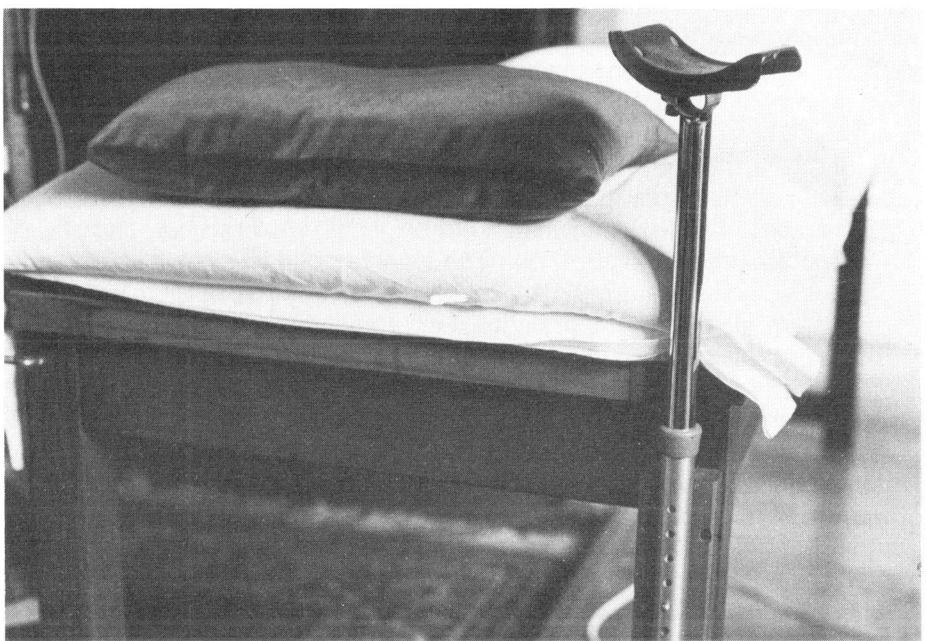

Figure 59a.   Adaptation to examination couch for ACR taking.

that is a low area beneath the curve, corresponds to a decreased pulse wave occurring after the dicrotic notch, and this indicates a negative ACR, and conversely, a high integral indicates a positive ACR. This is seen in Figures 61 and 62 showing the ACR response on the equipment used by Navach.

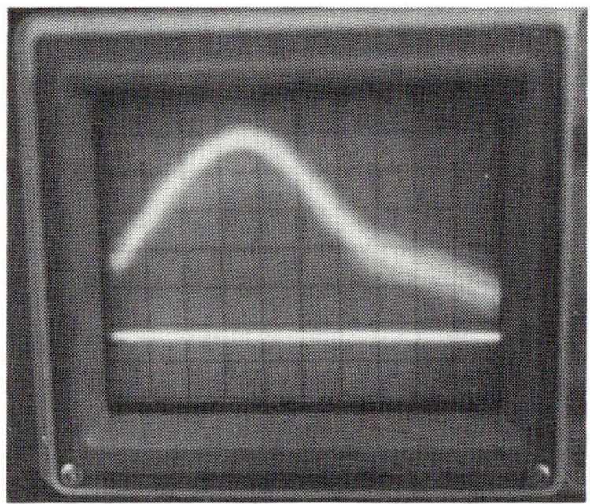

Figure 61.   A negative ACR with a low integral of the area after the dicrotic notch (see Appendix II).

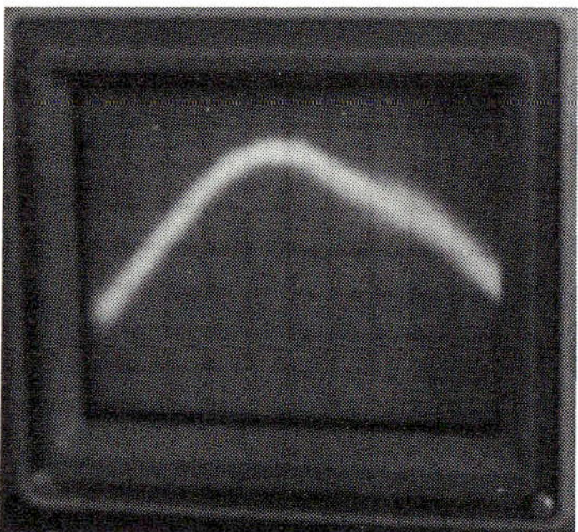

Figure 62.   A positive ACR with a high integral of the area after the dicrotic notch (see Appendix II)

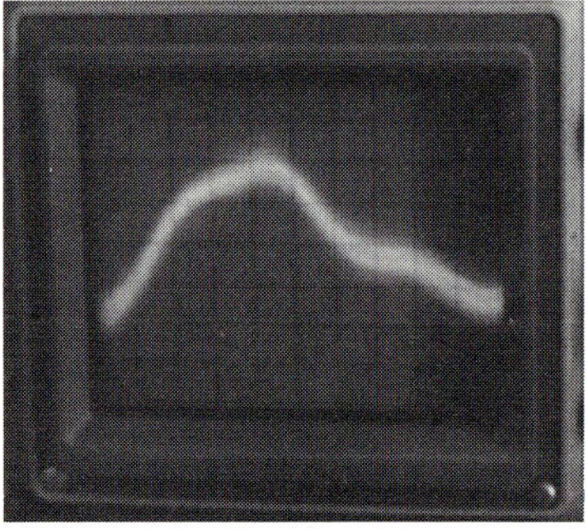

Figure 63.   Resting ACR curve taken from ACR recording apparatus made by Navach.

Navach has claimed to be able to quantitate the significance of an ACR by the angle at which the rising phase of the second half of the pulse complex occurring after the dicrotic notch occurs. A typical resting ACR curve in an average healthy subject has an angle of 25°.

An increase in the angle to 45° or more from the resting angle of 25° indicates a strong positive ACR, and a further increase of the angle is of increasing significance regarding the ACR response. Such a positive ACR response is shown in Figure 64.

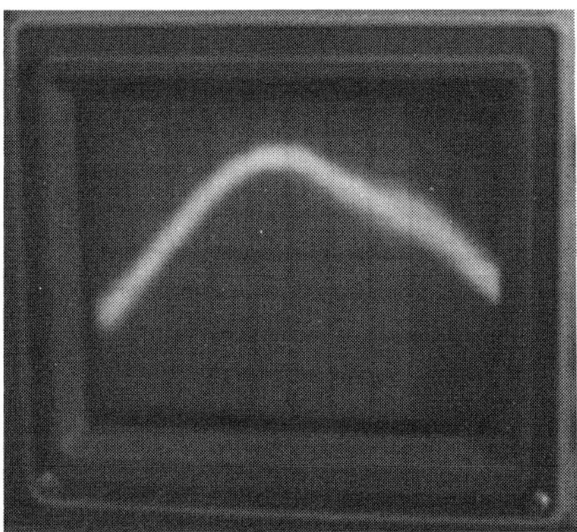

Figure 64.   A positive ACR taken from Navach's ACR reading apparatus.

If a pulse recording is made with a pulse sensor which records an initial positive deflection followed by a negative deflection, such as a typical pulse complex recorded by the electronic pulsograph (see section on Electronic Pulsography), then the part of the pulse wave occurring after the dicrotic notch corresponds to the area beneath the zero line on the electronic pulsograph recording. A full description of Navach's equipment and findings is given in Appendix II at the end of this section.

CHAPTER TEN

REFLEX ZONES OF THE AURICLE

Auricular medicine divides the auricle into seven zones each characterized by ACR response to a specific frequency of stimulation. For example if a frequency of five cycles per second (from a source such as a flashing light) is applied to the ear, a positive ACR will be produced by this stimulation over the concha, but over no other zones on the ear with this particular frequency.

According to the somatotopic mapping of the ear, the concha corresponds to the abdomen, but if this same frequency of five cycles per second is applied to abdominal skin only areas of skin overlying diseased organs give a positive ACR. For instance, if there is gall bladder disease, then the area over the right hypochondrium will produce a positive ACR if this area of skin is searched with an energy source emitting five cycles per second. This has obvious diagnostic uses.

Similarly the other six areas of the auricle have been particularized according to their ACR response, and this is shown in Figure 65. The area corresponding to the particular frequency zone is judged to have a similar resonant frequency to the equivalent area on the ear. This is illustrated in the same diagram.

Each of these resonant frequencies can be represented by a colour, and Nogier has worked out a series of seven colour filters, each corresponding to a particular frequency zone. The Wratten number of each filter is listed in Figure 65. In auricular medicine a set of seven colour filters, together with an eighth filter which contains a small section of each of the seven colours, is often used, and is to be regarded as an essential piece of equipment when practising auricular therapy* (Figure 66).

If a light is shone through the appropriate colour filter, as in Figure 67, and directed onto the ear zone to which the colour corresponds a positive ACR will occur.

A torch with a revolving turret with windows made from each of the colour filters corresponding to the seven frequency zones can be used for this purpose† (Figure 68).

*Colour programme. Series of eight colour filters produced by Sedatelec, 135 Route Neuve, Irigny, France.
†Torch with revolving turret of six filters, either D2 series or D3 series. Available from Sedatelec (see Figure 68).

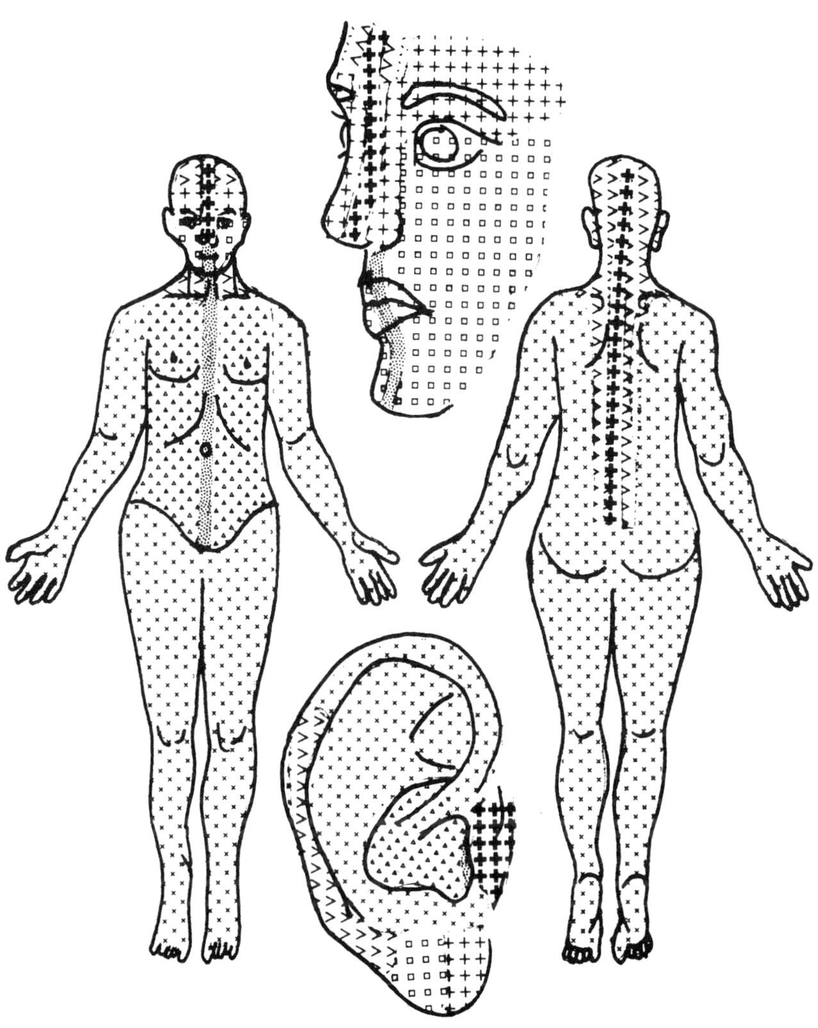

Note: Zone A is situated on the inner surface of the tragus.

= ZONE A (Kodak Wratten filter 22, 2.5hz)
= ZONE B (Kodak Wratten filter 25, 5hz)
= ZONE C (Kodak Wratten filter 4, 10hz)
= ZONE D (Kodak Wratten filter 23A, 20hz)
= ZONE E (Kodak Wratten filter 44, 40hz)
= ZONE F (Kodak Wratten filter 98, 80hz)
= ZONE G (Kodak Wratten filter 30,160hz)

Figure 65.   Frequency zones of the ear and their resonant frequencies together with somatic correspondences (after Nogier).

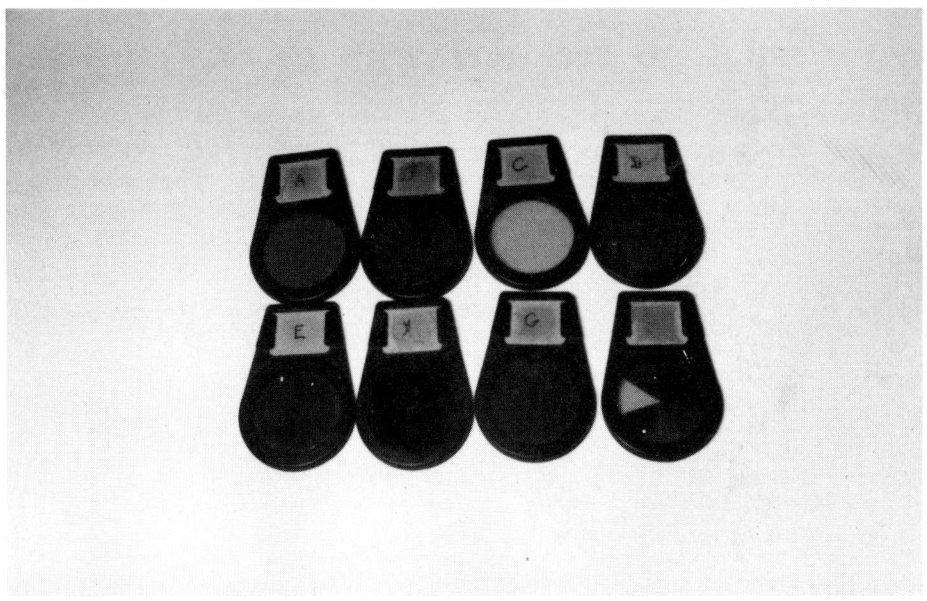

Figure 66.   The seven colour programme consisting of seven individual filters and one filter containing all seven colours.

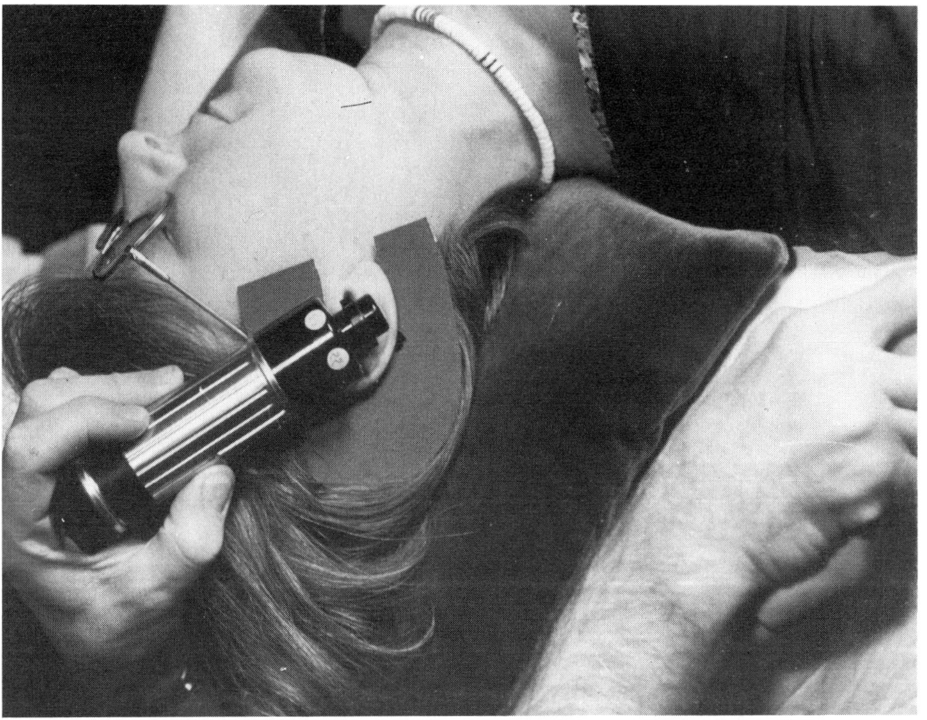

Figure 67.   Coloured light being shone onto the ear using a torch with a revolving turret.

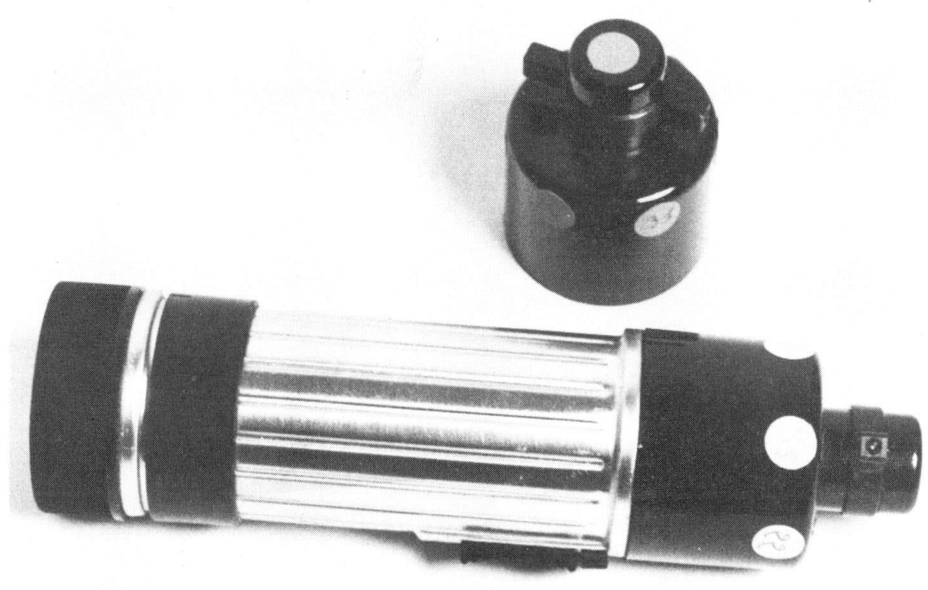

Figure 68. Torch with revolving turret, each window containing a coloured filter.

A useful exercise for any practitioner new to auricular therapy is, having first mastered the ACR, to then examine the ear with the relevant coloured light, using the revolving turret torch, and confirm that the particular areas of the ear give positive ACRs in response to their resonant colour, which is effectively the same as applying a specific frequency onto that zone of the ear, i.e. a frequency or a colour both correspond to a particular energy level.

The concept of specific ear zones resonating at particular frequencies is of use in auricular therapy, and from the observations of many practitioners the division of the ear into seven zones appears to be correct, although it has to be admitted that as yet there has been no scientifically acceptable method of demonstrating this in an experimental situation, so the concept remains very much a practical concept, awaiting scientific investigation should such a method yield itself.

Navach's equipment for recording the ACR would be one possible way of investigating this (see Appendix).

Laterality

Laterality is an ill defined, but clinically important, concept in auricular therapy. Nogier claims that poorly lateralized patients respond badly to therapies of all sorts, and that particularly in auricular therapy the patient's laterality, or lack of it, ought to be determined and put right if incorrect prior to any treatment.

The concept of laterality is a complex one. The idea that laterality is important in chronic pain for example has been suggested by Merskey[1] Merskey noted that pain was more often lateralized to the left, except in cases of trigeminal neuralgia. No reason for this was given. Merskey also noted that hysterical conversion of symptoms are also more common on the left. He then states that experimental evidence implies that the right hemisphere is less efficient than the left in processing cutaneous sensory input, and concludes by claiming that neurological and psychiatric studies support the view that the right hemisphere is dominant for emotional experience, and this may help to determine the left-sided preponderance of pain. Not surprisingly, Merskey's paper was soon challenged with opposite claims by Hall, Hayward and Chapman[2] So clearly the subject remains controversial. With this in mind however, the concept of laterality, as taught by Nogier, is clinically useful even though it remains a subject of debate. Auricular medicine describes a legion of methods, mostly using colour filters, but in some cases using other equipment, in order to determine laterality. For the newcomer to auricular medicine this can be confusing, and as all the methods are defining the same thing it is only necessary to learn one method for determining laterality. The method used by the author will be described, and at least it has the merit of being simple, quick and easy to perform.

First, filter B from the colour programme is placed on sympathetic skin (such as forearm skin), and then zone B (concha) is palpated with a pressure palpator, first on one side and then on the other. On the side to which the patient is lateralized, that is the right concha for a right hander and the left concha for a left hander, then on that side, and on that side only, a positive ACR should be obtained whilst using the pressure palpator with filter B on the forearm. On the non-dominant side no ACR should be obtained. If an equal ACR is obtained both sides, and this is the most common abnormality, or if the laterality is switched, i.e. a positive ACR is obtained on the non-dominant side, then a diagnosis of disordered laterality is made. Similarly any other colour filter could be used; for example if filter C is put on sympathetic skin, instead of probing the concha (zone B) the area representing zone C lying between the anti-helix and the helix should be palpated. It is interesting to try this exercise without the colour filter applied to the skin of the forearm, on doing this no difference is recorded from one side to the other, and often no ACR is perceived. The placing of the colour filter on the skin must be having some overall affect, which is difficult to believe but always occurs in practice. The reasons for this are unknown, although many auricular therapists have a large number of possible explanations, all of which are notable for their lack of credibility.

Another method for determining laterality will be outlined in a later chapter.

Inversion The main abnormality occurring in any auricle is an instability of laterality, as just described. Another less common abnormality is so-called 'inversion'. In inversion it is assumed that the sympathetic skin is reacting as if it were parasympathetic, and that the parasympathetic skin is reacting as if it were sympathetic. The way to detect this is again, to use either a B or a C filter; for example a B filter is placed on the forearm, and then the torch with the revolving turret is used, with the B filter in place, and this is shone over the B zone on the ear, i.e. the concha. If a positive ACR is detected over zone B with a B filter on sympathetic skin, this indicates that the auricle is not showing inversion. If no positive ACR is noted when shining the torch through B filter on the concha, but instead a positive ACR is noted when shining the B filter on C zone, which is the sympathetic part of the ear, then this indicates that inversion is present. Similarly the same procedure can be performed using the C filter on the periphery and shining the torch through the C filter onto the C zone of the ear, and noting if a positive ACR occurs. If it does, then no inversion is present; if not, and instead a positive ACR with a C filter shone on the ear is produced through shining this on B zone, then inversion is present. This has to be corrected before therapy is attempted, and methods for doing this will be outlined in a later chapter.

It is difficult to accept that placing a colour filter on the skin produces any change, but when one uses the technique as described for detecting laterality, first with the filter on the skin, and then without the filter, different reactions of the ACR are obtained. This would indicate that the colour filter is having some sort of an effect. **The Use of Colour Filters**

If the ACR is palpated and either the white or the black side of the so-called black/white hammer* is passed over the auricle above the skin, then multiple ACRs will be noted (see Figure 69). If the colour filters are then placed on the forearm, for example the colour filter containing all the seven colours and the ACR is palpated again, and the ear searched again by passing either the black or the white side of the black/white hammer close to the ear but not touching the skin, instead of obtaining a large number of ACRs only a small number are detected, and this small number of ACRs are generally more easily detected (see Figure 69). Nogier explains this by using an analogy with the tuning of a radio set, in that if the programme is not tuned correctly then background noise is present. If the background noise is tuned out, then the programme comes through loud and clear.

It would appear that placing the seven colour programme on the forearm skin, or indeed any colour referring to any zone of the ear, if that zone is going to be searched, i.e. colour filter B for zone B etc., has the same affect as tuning the radio, and it therefore 'lowers background noise'. This can be confirmed repeatedly in the clinical situation. The reason that the seven colour programme is most effective for this purpose is that it includes all the major ear frequencies within it. The points which then 'stand out' over the ear (that is those points which produce a positive ACR, when a black or a white tip from the black/white hammer is passed over the auricle) are the points which require treatment.

The application of filters and their use in auricular therapy is a fruitful area both for diagnosis and therapy. The use of filters in auricular therapy has tended to become over-complex. Much of this complexity consists of detail which is perhaps correct but not necessarily useful; in other words there are many ways of detecting laterality instability by the use of various combinations of filters, not only using colour filters, but polaroid filters, drug filters etc. All of these methods produce the same answer, but in the author's opinion, to avoid confusion, it is only necessary to learn, at the most, two methods for detecting any particular situation on the ear. Therefore the author has attempted to minimize the detail given in relationship to the use of filters in auricular medicine.

In summary filters in auricular medicine are used to aid in the detection of points which need treating. They can be regarded as tuning devices. The choice of filter in many ways depends not only on one's knowledge of auricular medicine, but also on that of allopathic physiology and pharmacology. This will become clearer later when the use of drug filters will be discussed.

*Black/White hammer manufactured by Sedatelec, 135 Route Neuve, Irigny, France.

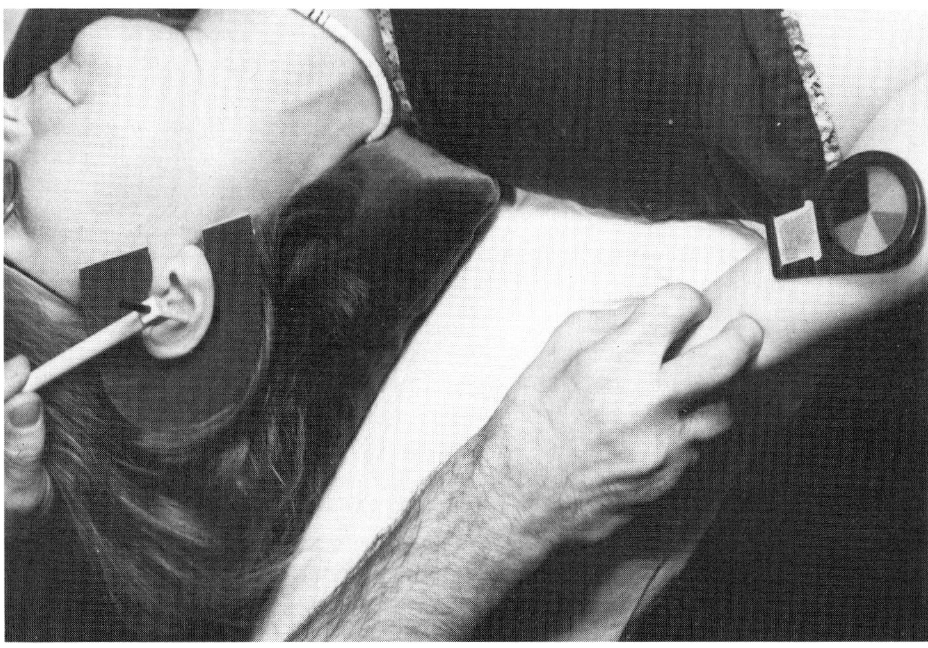

Figure 69.   Point detection using a black/white hammer with the seven colour filter on the forearm.

Biotic Points In order to make pathological points stand out more clearly the appropriate filters are placed on sympathetic skin. If the filters are placed on parasympathetic skin, i.e. skin above the clavicles excluding zone C of the ear, or the sacral parasympathetics, then different points become detectable. These points are termed 'biotic points' by Nogier, and he claims that these points refer to deep underlying pathology. The practical application of this is that by detecting and treating biotic points the results of ear acupuncture treating pathological points, having first placed the filter on sympathetic skin (i.e. the forearm) can be improved on. This can be a useful adjunct to therapy of pathological points.

Specific Use of Each Colour Filter Nogier teaches that each colour filter can be used to detect specific groups of disorders, and from a practical point of view it is useful to know these associations. The author finds the information concerned with filters A, B, C & E to be of clinical use. The associations given for filters D, F & G are in the author's opinion not of much clinical use, though they may be correct.

Filter A

This is useful for detecting IgGa and IgM mediated immunity. The way to detect this is to palpate the ACR and pass filter A from parasympathetic skin to sympathetic skin. This is generally done by putting filter A over the forehead and passing it over onto the sympathetic zone of the ear (this corresponds to zone C). If a positive ACR is obtained when filter A arrives over sympathetic skin, then this means that an allergy is present. This test is a useful preliminary before teating a patient for food sensitivity. In a patient with no allergies no positive ACR should be noted when filter A is put over the forehead or over the sympathetic part of the ear.

Filter B

This filter can be used in the detection of alimentary and abdominal disturbances. In order to detect a diseased area in the abdomen filter B can be passed over the abdomen whilst feeling the patient's pulse. A positive ACR will be detected over the skin overlying a diseased organ.

Filter C

This is useful for diseases of the locomotor system such as arthritis.

Filter D

This filter can be used to detect disturbances in communication between the right and left side of the brain, i.e. the corpus callosum. This is important in poor or reversed laterality.

Filter E

Filter E is useful for detecting IgE mediated immunity such as is seen in immediate hypersensitivity reactions. This sort of reaction is typified by the patient who eats shellfish or strawberries and within minutes comes out in an urticarial skin eruption. This filter is used to detect this sort of reaction in exactly the same way as filter A, i.e. filter E is passed from the parasympathetic skin (forehead) onto sympathetic skin (area C of the auricle). If a positive ACR is perceived when the filter arrives over the sympathetic area of the ear, then IgE mediated immunity is present.

On the ear homunculus, area E corresponds to the spinal cord, therefore this filter may also be used for defining diseased areas of the spinal cord, i.e. in cases of disseminated sclerosis.

Filter F

This area defines the subcortical structures such as the brain stem and thalamus. Zone F nearly always yields a pathological point in chronic pain, presumably because the thalamus mediates pain input.

Filter G

This represents the higher cortical centres, and zone G on the ear often needs treating in psychiatric illness.

CHAPTER ELEVEN

DETECTION OF PATHOLOGICAL POINTS ON THE EAR

Pathological points on the ear can be detected by a variety of different methods:

    (a)   Pressure Palpation
    (b)   Electrical Point Detection
    (c)   Black/White Hammer
    (d)   Positive/Negative Hammer
    (e)   Gold/Silver Hammer

The detection of pathological points using the pressure palpator, and also the use of an electrical point detector (i.e. the *Punctoscope*) have been described in detail in Chapter 1. The other three methods mentioned all depend on the use of the ACR. Each hammer consists of a shaft with a crosspiece at the top; one end of the crosspiece being either black or white, gold or silver, positive or negative. A black/white hammer, positive/negative and gold/silver hammer are illustrated in Figure 69.

Each combination, i.e. black/white, gold/silver or positive/negative are to be understood as energy levels; black, for example, being low and white high in energy. Perhaps in this case the chief role is probably played by the light absorption characteristics of black (maximal light absorption), and white (minimal light absorption). Gold and silver can be regarded as having different electrode potentials, silver having an electrode potential of $+0.8$ volts, and gold $+1.68$ volts. An increased difference in electrode potential can be obtained by using a metal lower down in the electrochemical series than silver, for example zinc with an electrode potential of -0.76 volts. Zinc can be easily obtained by dismantling an ordinary Tricell battery, zinc forming the outer coating (negative plate) of the battery. In clinical practice the use of the gold/silver hammer provides satisfactory results, and in this sense gold is higher in energy than silver.

The positive/negative hammer can be understood as being similar to the gold/silver hammer in that there is a difference in potential between one side and the other, i.e. the positive side is at a higher potential than the negative side. Generally speaking a 9 volt hammer is used. It is interesting to note that if a high voltage

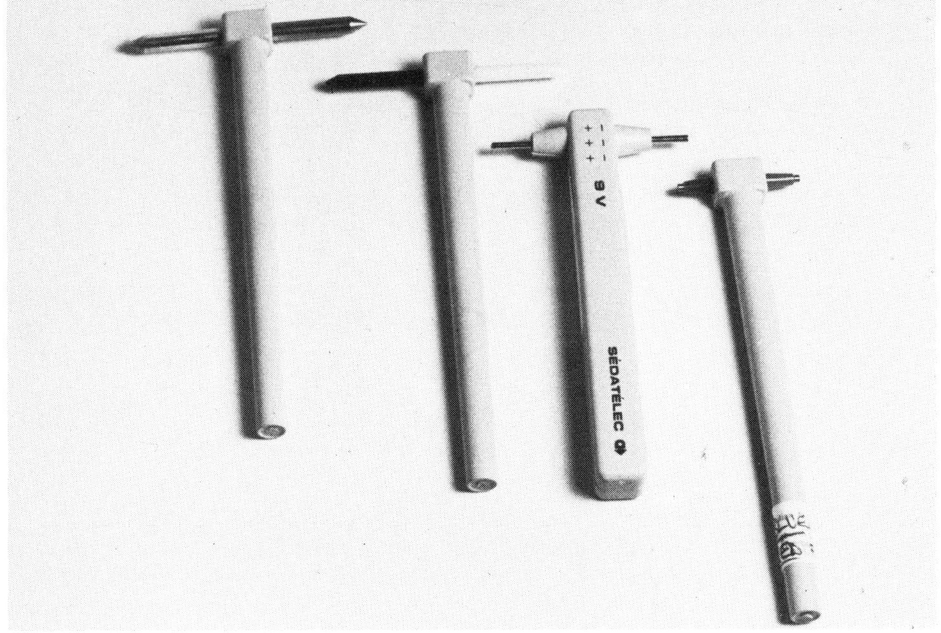

Figure 70. Various hammers used for point detection. From left to right: gold/silver hammer; black/white hammer; positive/negative hammer; bar magnet with north pole on the left side (coloured blue) and south pole on the right side (coloured red).

hammer is used (in practice this means something over 18 volts), instead of giving a positive ACR over a pathological point a negative ACR may be produced. This is probably the same phenomenon as is obtained when shining a very bright light over sympathetic skin. Initially, when the light is at medium intensity, a positive ACR is produced, but as the intensity of applied energy is increased the ACR becomes negative (see Chapter 9). This phenomenon can be easily confirmed, by using a 27 volt hammer, which can be made by joining three-volt batteries in series and using the appropriate lead from each end of the series of three cells attached to the crossbar of the positive/negative hammer. Therefore, the 9 volt hammer is found to be the right voltage level for a positive ACR to occur over a pathological point.

The Use of Point Detection 'Hammers' in Order to Detect Pathological Points

The first step in order to detect pathological points is to use some system of eliminating 'background noise' by the use of a filter. A seven colour programme could be used as explained in the previous chapter. Some practitioners consider that earthing the patient is necessary.[1] This can be accomplished by using a short length of copper piping, together with a wire connection to the earth of the mains supply. In the author's view earthing the patient by asking him to hold the copper cylinder in one hand is necessary when working near to power lines, or in any institution where equipment such as X-ray apparatus is situated in the same building. The claim that an earth needs to be held by the patient in each hand has not been confirmed by the author, and a single copper cylinder with the patient holding this

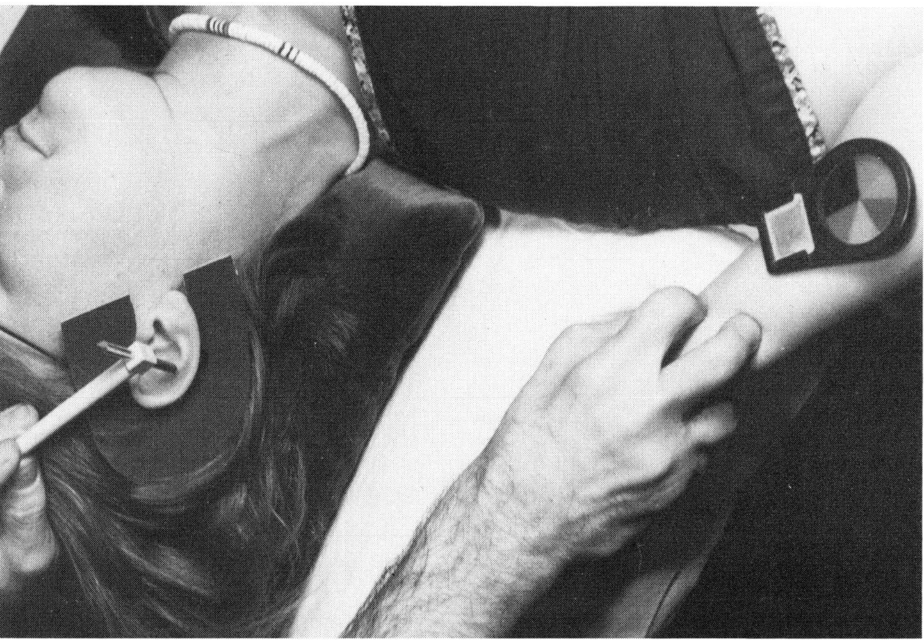

Figure 71.   Point detection on the ear using a gold/silver hammer.

in either hand is found to be satisfactory in practice.

A seven colour programme is placed on sympathetic skin (i.e. the forearm); the ACR is palpated, and whilst one thumb is left on the radial pulse in order to palpate the ACR on one side, on the other side the hammer is slowly and carefully passed over each zone of the ear. A number of pathological points will generally be detected either with one or the other side of whichever hammer is used. The tip of the hammer should be slowly moved over the surface of the ear, holding the tip of the hammer some quarter-inch or so above the skin. Touching the skin of the ear whilst using a point of detection method making use of the ACR confuses the picture. This is hard to believe but in practice is the only method which produces an obvious result in terms of a positive ACR response (see Figures 71 and 72).

In order to understand what may be happening when point detecting with these various hammers, using the ACR as an indication of positive response, the acupuncture point has to be conceived as being similar in many respects to a battery. This is an almost identical concept to that outlined in the section on 'Electro-acupuncture According to Voll' in Volume I. In electrical terms what may be wrong with the battery-like acupuncture point is that it may be too highly charged (therefore too high in energy) or too poorly charged (therefore low in energy). Therefore, if a high energy source is passed over a pathological point which is too low in energy, a positive ACR response will occur; in other words the body will respond positively to a stimulus which has a tendency to restore that point to normality. This high energy source therefore corresponds to the gold side of the gold/silver hammer, or the positive side of the positive/negative hammer, and also the black side of the black/white hammer. The opposite pertains to point detection over a point high in energy. This means that a point low in energy requires a gold needle in order to

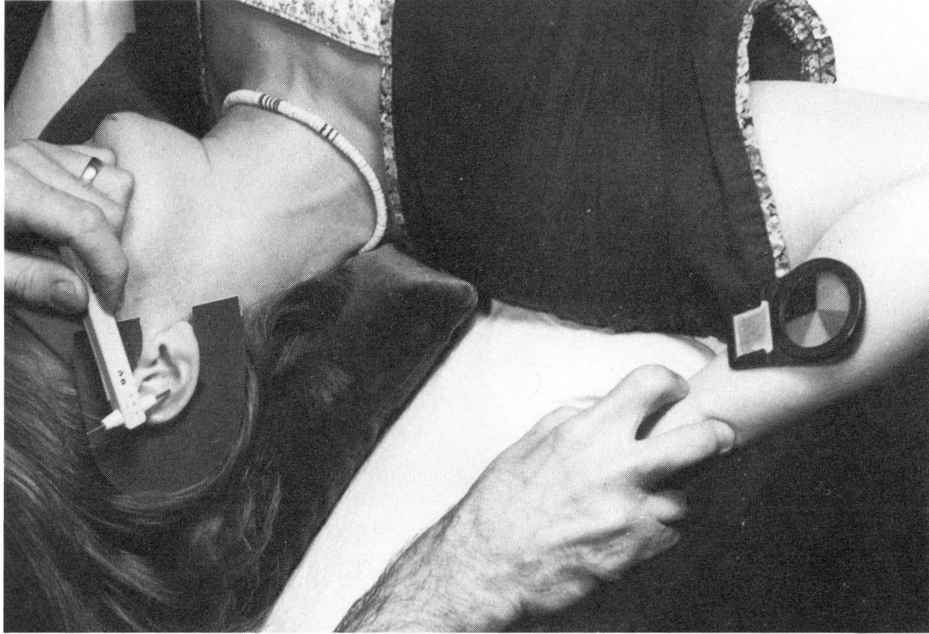

Figure 72. Point detection on the ear using a positive/negative hammer.

raise its energy level, and will give a positive ACR to the black side of the black/white hammer, the positive side of the positive/negative hammer and to the gold side of the gold/silver hammer, the opposite pertains for a point high in energy which needs discharging, and therefore treatment with a silver needle.

So in summary:

BLACK, POSITIVE, AND GOLD ARE ALL SYNONYMOUS IN ENERGY TERMS. THIS EQUALS TREATMENT WITH A GOLD NEEDLE.

WHITE, NEGATIVE AND SILVER ARE ALL SYNONYMOUS IN ENERGY TERMS. THIS EQUALS TREATMENT WITH A SILVER NEEDLE.

A magnet may also be used for point detection, and a north pole corresponds to the positive side of the positive/negative hammer, and therefore with gold and black. The south pole corresponds to the negative side of the positive/negative hammer, and therefore with the silver and white. (This relationship of the magnetic poles to the positive/negative hammer is derived from the basic laws of electro-magnetism).

The idea that an ACR response can be elicited by passing an object near to the skin without touching the skin stretches credibility to say the least. However, it has been a consistently observed phenomena by practitioners using auricular medicine. Recently there has been some indication as to why this may be happening, and this has been provided by the original and innovative work of Dumitrescu.[?] Dumitrescu has shown that all biological systems are surrounded by a layer consisting of water vapour and ions of various sorts. He has termed this the 'proximal electric medium'. This extends out to approximately 2 inches from the skin of the human subject.

Dumitrescu has also shown, using a variety of imaging techniques, that the proximal electric medium is of major importance in subserving the function of energetic interchange between the body and its environment, and indeed Dumitrescu has shown it to be exceptionally sensitive to infinitesimal changes in electrical characteristics of the external environment in which the body is placed. Furthermore, he has discovered that over an acupuncture point ionic flows exist consisting predominantly of positive or negative ions, depending on whether the acupuncture point needs ions of one sort or another to correct its charge abnormality. This ionic flow has been shown to occur in a spiral fashion, coming out from the acupuncture point rather like a fountain. This would therefore explain why placing an object close to the skin without touching the skin will produce a change in the body's proximal electric medium. As to how this is perceived by the body remains an unanswered question. The fact that it is perceived in one form or another is practically beyond question. Striking evidence for this is provided in Dumitrescu's book *Electrographic Imaging in Medicine and Biology* (edited by the author), which outlines these effects in detail. In the author's view the explanation is most likely to be that the autonomic nervous system has an important and hitherto unrecognized afferent function, namely of responding in a sensory way to ambient electromagnetic fields. As the ACR is an autonomic phenomena, then this hypothesis would explain the physical signs as outlined here, and would also explain why the ACR can be used for allergy testing (see section on Clinical Ecology).

Up till the present time it has been disputed that man has any magnetic sense, although in evolutionary terms it would seem reasonable to think that as man has evolved on the earth, which can be likened to a magnet, then it is likely that he has also developed a magnetic sense. Recent evidence has been produced by Baxter[3] who has shown by means of clever experimentation that man does have a magnetic sense. The author's feeling is that all of these findings lend credibility to auricular medicine, and indeed to EAV and to acupuncture in general, and therefore provide a cogent reason as to why these disciplines need to be taken more seriously by mainstream medicine.

Generally speaking all the points detected in one autonomic zone of the ear, that is either the sympathetic or the parasympathetic zone, tend to show all the same abnormalities in electrical terms, i.e. all the points detected in the sympathetic zone of one ear will either all be highly charged, or all be poorly charged. The converse always occurs in the parasympathetic zone of the same ear. In practical terms, this means that if points requiring treatment with gold needles are found in the sympathetic zone of one ear, and if any points are detected in the concha of the same ear, then these points will almost certainly be found to require a silver needle. If this is not what is found then it is likely that the practitioner has made a mistake and he should go back and check. Very occasionally this general rule is found not to apply, and so if the same findings are made on rechecking then the initial findings were probably correct, and perhaps gold and silver points are present in either one sympathetic or parasympathetic zone.

The same principle of opposite needling, i.e. silver instead of gold or gold instead of silver, is noted when searching the same zone of the opposite ear. For example, if gold points are detected on the sympathetic zone of the right ear, and if pathological points are found on the sympathetic zone of the left ear, then invariably, these points will be found to be silver points, and vice versa. Therefore the change in polarity of points not only occurs from sympathetic to parasympathetic zones on the same side, but also applies to homologous areas from one side of the body to the other. This coherence in energy levels of pathological points has been noted by the author, and does not seem to have been generally recognized as yet by Nogier or by any of the doctors teaching Nogier's method in Germany or France. This coherence of polarity is in line with Manaka's[4] ideas of the body being divided into quadrants in terms of energy. Manaka states that energy zones change from side to side and from back to front, the dividing lines being the Dumo and the Renmo (representing the posterior and anterior midline respectively) and also the lateral midline of the body, representing the division between front and back.

It will be clear whether the point needs treating with a good or a silver needle, even though the point will give some reaction to the opposite metal (or the opposite side of the detection hammer). Generally this reaction will be not as strong as when using the side of the hammer indicating the needle required in order to treat that point. If it is impossible to be sure what metal to use, then stainless steel needles should be tried or the principle of different metals should be applied as outlined above. In other words, if silver points are detected in the right concha, and then pathological points are detected on the sympathetic zone of the same ear, but it is unclear as to whether these points need to be treated in silver or in gold, then having found silver points in the concha of the same ear, it is probable that the points in the sympathetic zone of the same ear will require treatment with gold.

One important exception to the rule of opposite needling in terms of gold and silver from sympathetic to parasympathetic, and from side to side, is the case of the tragus. As stated in Chapter 7 the tragus represents midline structures and can be thought of as being bilaterally represented. Therefore there is no general rule as to which metal the tragus needs to be needled in.

When detecting points on the auricle it will often be found that points tend to lie along a line which may occur at any position across the ear, for example from top to bottom, or from front to back of the ear. The most common line along which points tend to occur is on a radius drawn out from point zero. The second most common line on which points occur is on a vertical line from top to bottom of the ear.

The pattern of points occurring in lines is by no means universal, but it is worth noting, as it can be useful to the beginner in auricular medicine.

Great care is required whilst searching the auricle for points which need treating. This means slow and careful searching with whichever hammer is chosen for point detection. On passing over the point the ACR will become positive and on passing away from the point it will become negative. This procedure can be repeated a number of times over each point to locate the exact centre of the point, then this should be marked with a felt tip pen. In order to obtain the best possible results with ear acupuncture absolute accuracy is essential, so painstaking point detection is required in order to achieve this end. The positive/negative hammer is the most useful method for point finding in painful conditions. In all other cases the

Practical Considerations When Detecting Pathological Ear Points

black/white hammer is satisfactory. The gold/silver hammer offers nothing more than the black/white or the positive/negative hammer, and as the gold/silver hammer is an expensive item it can usually be dispensed with, and satisfactory point detection, with determination of needle type to be used, can be carried out using the black/white hammer or the positive/negative hammer.

The Application of Filters in Point Detection The seven colour programme as a filter for point detection has already been described in detail. However, a wide variety of filters can be used and the points detected bear some relationship to the filter chosen. The seven colour programme should be regarded as a general filter for detection of pathological points. If a condition such as chronic pain is being treated, then an analgesic may be used as a filter; for example morphine. In practice a number of morphine ampoules in a transparent plastic container are placed on sympathetic skin, and a further ampoule is used to search round the ear, moving the ampoule over the ear in exactly the same manner as when using the positive/negative or black/white hammer. With this method once the point has been detected and marked with a felt tip pen, further detection with a black/white hammer or a positive/negative hammer etc., needs to be carried out in order to determine whether the point needs a gold or a silver needle. In other words, when using a drug as a filter the drug itself within an ampoule is used in order to detect the points, and this indicates where the pathological points are but does not indicate which metal the point needs. Therefore a further search with an appropriate hammer is necessary in order to determine this.

Depending on whether the filter is placed on the arm (sympathetic skin), or on the forehead (parasympathetic skin), different points are detected. This can be

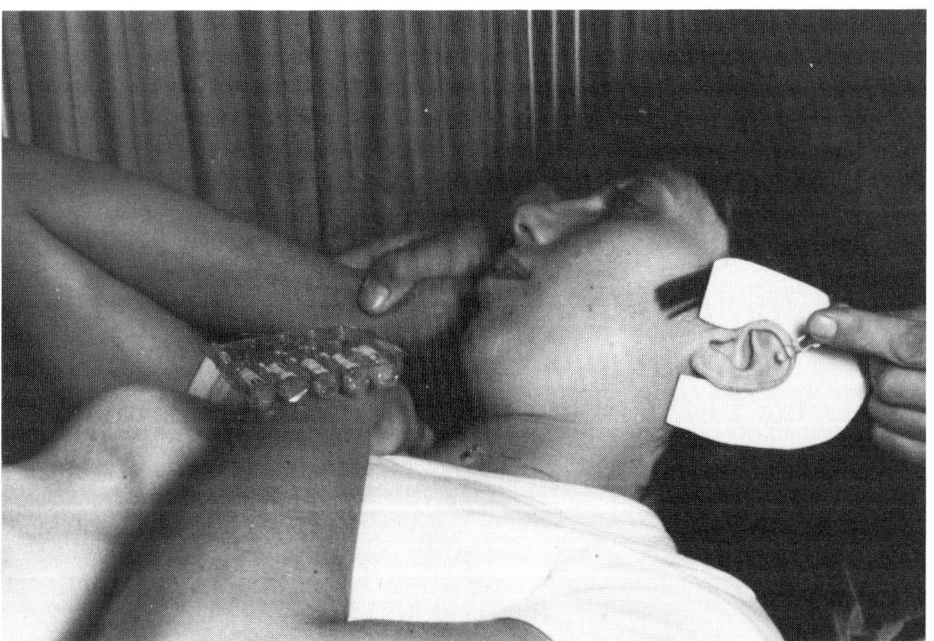

Figure 73. Point detection using morphine ampoules.

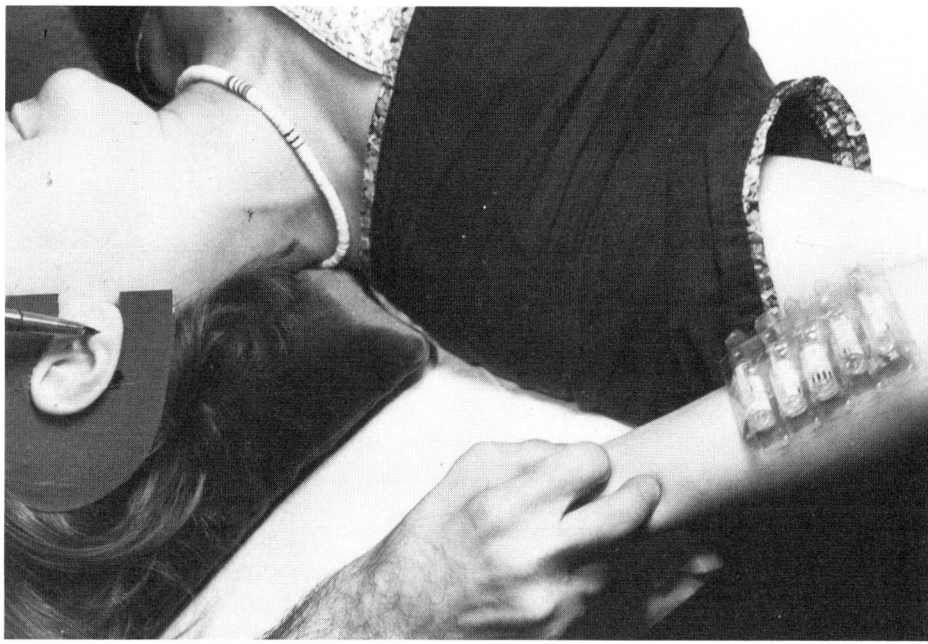

Figure 74.   Marking points detected with a felt tip pen.

confirmed by using firstly morphine ampoules as a filter placed on sympathetic skin in a patient with chronic pain, and then detecting pathological points on the ear using a morphine ampoule. This method of detection is shown in Figure 73. The pathological points are then marked with a felt tip pen (Figure 74), then the morphine ampoules are taken off sympathetic skin and placed on parasympathetic skin, i.e. the forehead. Then the ear is searched again using a morphine ampoule. On this occasion different points are found, and these should be marked with a different coloured felt tip pen. Following this Naloxone ampoules (Naloxone can be regarded as a pharmacological antagonist to morphine) are placed on sympathetic skin, then the ear is searched with a Naloxone ampoule. The points that were detected using morphine ampoules on the forehead are also detected if Naloxone is used as the filter on sympathetic skin. The converse also applies, i.e. the points that 'lit up' with morphine on the forearm (sympathetic skin) will be identical to those detected with Naloxone as a filter on the forehead. This is an important experiment as two practical conclusions can be drawn from it. The first is that different points 'light up' on the ear depending on which substance is used as a filter, and in theory the choice of filters is infinite, but in practice relies on the pharmacological knowledge of the practitioner. The second conclusion is that placing a drug on sympathetic skin is equivalent, in terms of points on the ear, to giving the patient the drug. Therefore, in a patient with pain, if these points are treated appropriately then the pain will disappear. If, however, the points are treated which 'light up' with morphine placed on the patient's forehead (i.e. on parasympathetic skin) then the pain does not disappear, and therefore placing a drug on parasympathetic skin can be taken as equivalent to removing the drug from the patient. In this case removing morphine from a patient with chronic pain can be visualized as something which will have no effect on the pain, and perhaps may make the pain worse. Therefore:

PLACING A DRUG FILTER ON SYMPATHETIC SKIN = A PATIENT REACTION AS IF THE DRUG WERE BEING GIVEN.

PLACING A DRUG FILTER ON PARASYMPATHETIC SKIN = A PATIENT REACTION AS IF THE DRUG WAS BEING TAKEN AWAY.

For detection of pain points any analgesic can be used as a filter, and also Noradrenaline can be useful. In the author's practice Noradrenaline is generally chosen. An obvious example in the choice of drug filter used is when using auricular medicine in the treatment of climacteric disorders. In this case the choice is of Oestrogen and Progesterone, either as combination tablets (the contraceptive pill); or as separate preparations. For this any equivalent drug preparation may be used, but prior to its use any tablet coating has to be removed and the substance of the tablet alone used for the filter. If an Oestrogen/Progesterone filter is placed on sympathetic skin, then points can be detected on the ear in the normal way.

It is possible to short-cut the procedure of searching with a tablet of the same substance, as that used for the previously described filters, as this can be cumbersome and certainly not as easy as searching with an ampoule. In these circumstances the author's practice is to use a black/white hammer for detecting points, as this will also indicate the choice of needle for the point detected. The author has found this method effective for climacteric problems and to be more rapidly and more specifically effective than the use of classical acupuncture in the same situation.

The method of using drug filters can be extended in order to treat habituation to tranquillizers. Often drug habituation responds well to ear acupuncture using points detected with the drug of habituation used as a filter placed on sympathetic skin, and the ear points detected treated appropriately. In the author's experience this form of therapy is more specific and generally more effective than the use of neuro-electric therapy. Neuro-electric therapy remains more effective when treating the more common addictions such as nicotine, alcoholism and hard drug addiction, although in these cases auricular therapy can be used as an adjunct using the drug of addiction as a filter placed on sympathetic skin.

A good example of the use of a drug as a filter placed on parasympathetic skin is post-pill anovulation in which case the anovulatory situation can be considered as possibly being related to longterm use of the Oestrogen/Progesterone contraceptive pill. Therefore, in order to correct the situation, the pill has to be 'removed' in order for ovulation to occur. Therefore the pill previously used by the patient can be used as a filter placed on parasympathetic skin. When using the contraceptive pill as a filter it is important to remove the coating. Then the points which are detected using the ACR can be needled appropriately. In the author's practice this has produced ovulation within a few hours of needling in a number of cases, and pregnancy has resulted. On one occasion a twin pregnancy resulted. Neither the patient nor the spouse had any family history of twinning. It must be emphasized that this cannot be regarded as a blanket treatment for infertility, but only for particular sorts of infertility, i.e. anovulation following longterm use of the contraceptive pill. This illustrates the principle of drug filters, and practitioners can devise their own drug filters depending on the clinical situation.

In conclusion any practitioner will soon become adept at sensible selection of filters for detection of points. If a choice of drug filter is not obvious, then the seven colour programme can be used as a filter and this may be regarded as a general filter. However, the drug filters, if correctly chosen, often give more specific and better results. In painful conditions Noradrenaline or any other analgesic are ideal filters for point detection.

CHAPTER TWELVE

THE TREATMENT OF PATHOLOGICAL POINTS

Pathological points on the ear can be treated in a number of different ways. The previous chapter referred to the use of gold and silver needles. The effect of a gold needle is supposed to tonify a point, or in electrical terms to charge the point up. The effect of a silver needle is to do the opposite. This effect of charging or discharging a point can be achieved with a magnet; the equivalent of charging up a point would be the use of a North pole; similarly, a South pole would have the opposite effect.

The application of magnets to the treatment of pathological points is made use of in the *Therapuncteur — EMS 20*. This equipment will be described in detail, as will the application of lasers to the treatment of pathological points. Laser energy is simply another way of treating a pathological point. Lastly, stainless steel needles may be used to treat pathological points; the use of this has been outlined in Chapter 8. The use of stainless steel needles must be regarded as the most unsophisticated method for treating pathological points.

In order to get a longer lasting effect a semi-permanent needle may be used. The use of semi-permanent needles and their insertion has been outlined in Chapter 8. In the first-aid situation, for example in toothache, then simply massaging the painful ear point is often enough to relieve pain. This generally will not have a long-lasting effect.

The methods for deciding whether a gold or a silver needle needs to be used, or by inference, as to whether North pole (positive) or South pole (negative) needs to be used etc., have been outlined in detail in the previous chapter.

Method of Needle Insertion   Having determined where the needles ought to be placed, and as to which sort of needle is required at each point detected, the patient's ACR is palpated with one hand and the point is approached with the needle in the opposite hand. The nearer the tip of the needle is to the centre of the point then the stronger the ACR becomes, until when the tip of the needle is directly over the centre of the point the ACR is maximal. The best method of being sure of 'hitting the centre of the point' is to

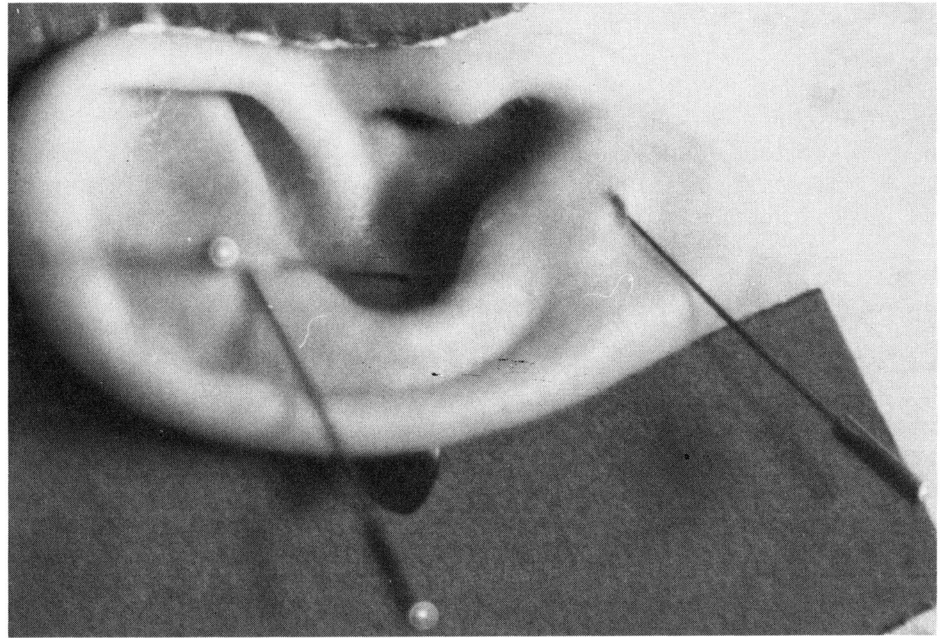

Figure 75.   Gold and silver needles in place on the ear.

pass the tip of the needle slowly over the point previously marked with a felt tipped pen, and note where the ACR appears maximal. Then, pass the needle over a line 90° to the first pass made with the needle, and again noting where the ACR appears maximal.

The point of intersection of these two imaginery lines is where the needle should be inserted. Absolute accuracy in the placement of the needles is essential in auricular therapy, and can make all the difference between getting a clinical result and having no effect at all. The needles should be inserted so that they support their own weight when using the rigid gold and silver needles as supplied by Sedatelec* This is illustrated in Figure 75. Finer gold and silver needles are available and these are less uncomfortable for the patient. On no account should the needles be inserted right through the auricle, although this method has been taught by some practitioners of auricular medicine. In the author's view this is a dangerous practice and can give rise to the immediate problem of haemorrhage, and the longer term problem of local infection at the needle site.

In clinical practice it is best to use a minimum number of needles as usually a more coherent result will be obtained. Try and limit the number of needles used on any one ear to a maximum of five. The needles should be left in place for approximately five minutes; leaving them in for any longer when using gold and silver needles doesn't seem to add any further beneficial effect. Stainless steel needles need to be left in longer, generally between ten to fifteen minutes. When using stainless steel needles the author's practice is to gently manipulate the needles. This follows the Chinese practice and is not taught in the French school of auricular

*Rigid gold and silver needles 32mm manufactured by Sedatelec. Fine gauge needles also available.

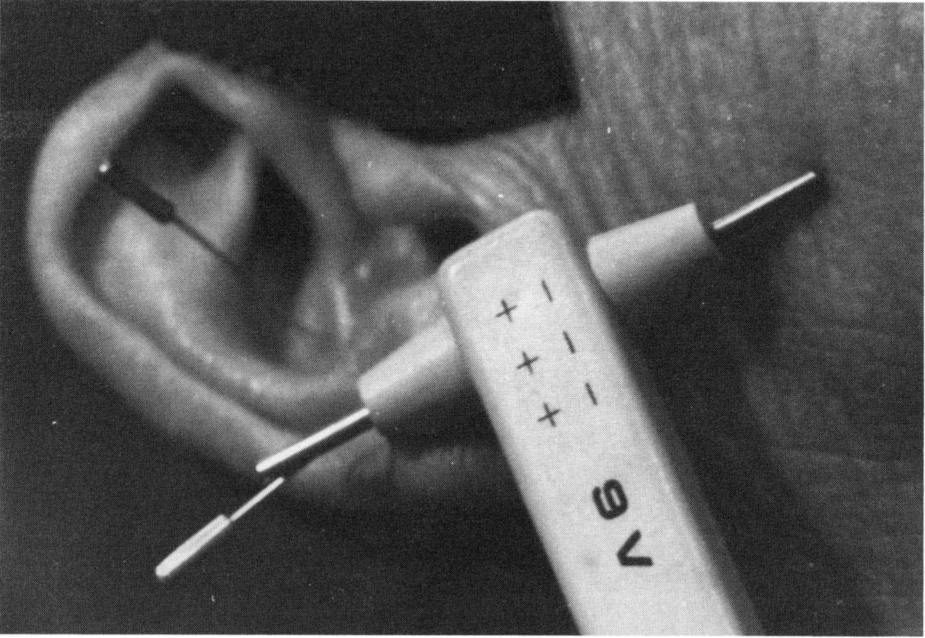

Figure 76.   Checking that needles are in the correct place using the positive/negative hammer.

therapy. When using gold and silver needles manipulation is not necessary, nor indeed desirable, as gold and silver needles are of a larger gauge than stainless steel needles and rotating these needles can be painful.

It is advisable to check whether the needles have been in place long enough, and the best method is to touch the handle of the needle with the appropriate side of the positive/negative hammer; for example if a gold needle is used then its handle, whilst in place, should be touched with the positive side of the positive/negative hammer (see Figure 76). If the needle is in the correct position, and has been in this place for sufficient time, then on touching the appropriate side of the positive/negative hammer against the handle of the needle the ACR should become negative. The ACR on a correctly placed needle becomes negative when applying this test after the needle has been in place for as little as one minute. If on touching the handle of the needle with the appropriate side of the positive/negative hammer the pulse either doesn't change, or a positive ACR is noted then this invariably means that the needle is in the wrong place. In this situation the needle should be withdrawn, and the point should be carefully searched again using the needle, feeling the ACR and re-inserting and checking to see whether the ACR has become negative on touching with the appropriate side of the positive/negative hammer.

A positive/negative hammer is the most useful hammer to use when checking if a needle is firstly in the correct place, and secondly has been in long enough. This is a useful check to make and beginners in auricular medicine will be surprised to find that initially a majority of the needles placed are in the wrong place. Often the correct place is only a distance of a millimeter or two away from the original incorrect placement. In the author's view this makes all the difference between success and failure in therapy. Nogier teaches that on needle insertion the patient should be asked to breathe in, and it is also commonly taught that when applying any filter to either sympathetic or parasympathetic skin, the patient should again be asked to breathe in. The reason for this advice is that autonomic tonus varies in inspiration and in expiration with the claim that parasympathetic tonality dominates during inspiration and that this is the best phase in which to either insert a needle or to place a filter on the skin. In the author's experience no clinically discernable difference is produced by either inserting a needle during inspiration or expiration, or by placing a filter on the skin during inspiration or expiration. If such an effect is present then the author's view is that it would be hard to prove it as statistically significant. Purists may well argue with this view and may wish to follow Nogier's teaching of always needling in inspiration, and also applying filters in inspiration.

Under no circumstances should electric current of any sort by applied to gold or silver needles. The normal rules for sterilization apply to gold or silver needles just as with stainless steel needles. Either they must be autoclaved in the normal fashion, making sure that gold and silver needles are not sterilized together, or alternatively, they may be sterilized by placing in surgical antiseptic solution for the time recommended by the manufacturers. A number of such solutions are available worldwide and are in standard use in operating theatres for quick sterilization of surgical instruments.

After the needles have been in this solution for the required period of time they can then be stored in absolute alcohol, again gold and silver needles should be kept separate from each other. The author's practice is to use two sets of Petri dishes,

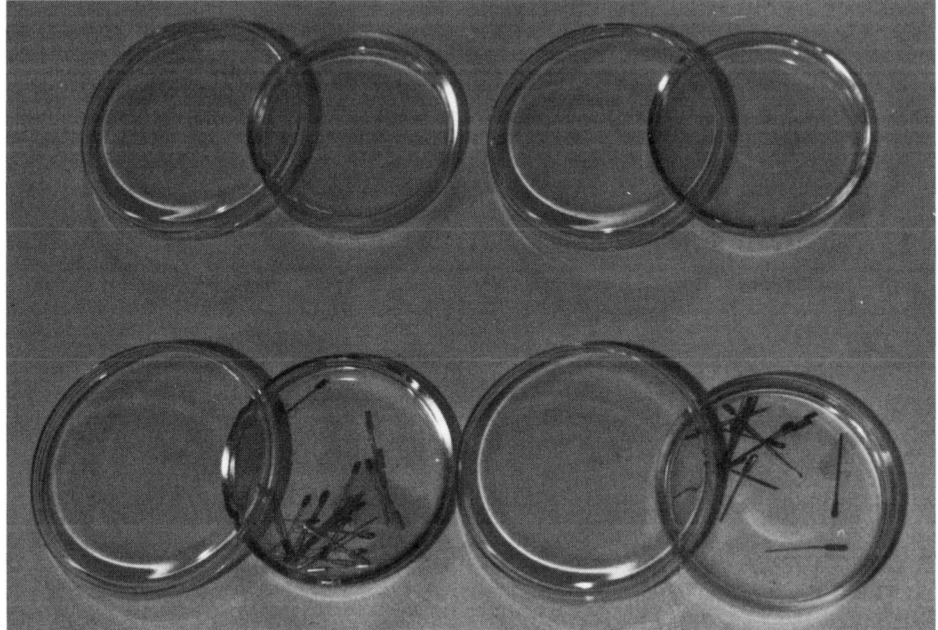

Figure 77. Petri dishes containing Cidex (upper dishes) and absolute alcohol (lower dishes).

one set containing an appropriate sterilizing solution, and the second set containing absolute alcohol (see Figure 77).

Frequency of Treatment　Patients are ideally treated weekly, just as with classical acupuncture. The response to treatment is identical to that of classical acupuncture in that a proportion of patients get initially worse, and for most clinical problems, a course of six treatments should be satisfactory. More complex problems will take longer, while simple problems may respond in one or perhaps two treatments. The author's practice is not to continue auricular therapy if no response is obtained after three treatments. It is useful to try different methods of stimulating points such as a laser or a magnetic field, as in some cases these have a more marked effect than using gold or silver needles. The indications for using lasers and magnetic fields will be discussed in a later chapter. There is no reason why ear acupuncture should not be combined with classical acupuncture; one can augment the effect of the other.

The Treatment of Disordered Laterality　The diagnosis of disordered laterality has been discussed in Chapter 10. The methods for correcting disordered laterality fall into two categories. One uses ear needles alone and the other concentrates on manipulation of the cervical spine. The exponents of each claim that their particular method is the most efficacious. In the author's experience manipulation of the spine at C7/T1 with lateral flexion towards the side of handedness, i.e. towards the right if a right-handed patient is being treated, and subsequent rotation away from the handed side, i.e. towards the left in a right-handed patient, is the most successful way of correcting disordered laterality. When using this method the physical signs as outlined in the test for laterality instability (see Chapter 10) always revert to normal. Nogier recommends this method of correction for disordered laterality, and claims that manipulation of C7/T1 junction affects the neck of the first rib and thereby the stellate ganglion which lies in this position. This claim is impossible to test, but from a practical point of view it works well. It is recommended that manipulation should only be carried out by practitioners competent in spinal manipulation. A number of textbooks on spinal manipulation are available, of which the author recommends the book by Bourdillion.[1] When contemplating manipulation to correct laterality instability it is important to know when not to manipulate, and as a rule of thumb the author recommends practitioners to bear in mind the following list of contraindications:

1. The possible existence of spinal secondaries, including conditions such as multiple myeloma.
2. Marked osteoporosis.
3. Patients with any significant boney deformity due to rheumatoid arthritis. A rupture of the transverse ligament of the atlas represents a significant problem here, and in the author's view only competent practitioners of spinal manipulation should attempt manipulation of 'rheumatoid' necks.

The German school of auricular therapy, headed by Bahr claims that instability of laterality can be adequately treated by the use of a silver pin placed in the position of the first rib, situated near to the anti-helix at the level of T1 on the dominant

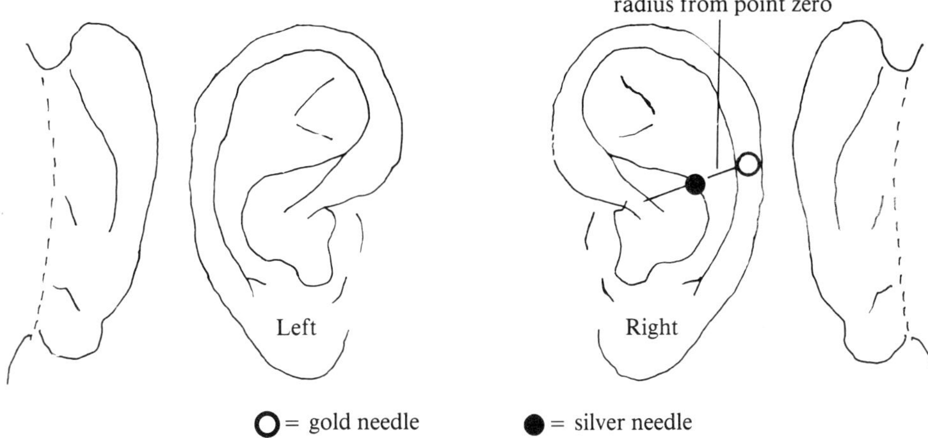

Figure 78.   Diagram showing needle placement for disordered laterality in a right-handed individual.

ear, using a silver needle, and a further needle, this time a gold needle, placed on the helix on the extremity of the radius drawn from point zero through the point of the first rib. This is illustrated in Figure 78.

This method corrects abnormal physical signs regarding unstable laterality. However, the effects are not as long lasting as when C7/T1 has been manipulated. In the author's experience only a gentle manipulation is required in order to produce long lasting effects; in other words the test for laterality remains normal on seeing the patient at the next appointment. When using needles for correcting laterality the laterality instability often recurrs. Correction of laterality is an important prerequisite to effective auricular therapy, so the author's practice is to always check for laterality instability, and then correct it prior to any treatment involving auricular therapy or auricular medicine.

Indications for Auricular Therapy

Auricular therapy may be used in any clinical situation in which classical acupuncture is useful. It may be used either on its own or as an adjunct to classical acupuncture. There are a number of clinical situations which are best treated using auricular therapy; it will therefore generally save time in these conditions to start therapy using auricular medicine. These conditions are:

(a) Neuralgias, such as Trigeminal Neuralgia, Post-herpetic Neuralgia, etc.
(b) Rheumatoid Arthritis.
(c) Autonomic Dystrophies.
(d) Root Pain.
(e) Therapy for drug habituation. For the treatment of hard drug addiction, nicotine or alcohol addictions, neuro-electric therapy is more effective than auricular medicine (see Volume I, Chapter 2).

CHAPTER THIRTEEN

THE THREE TISSUE LAYERS: THEIR ACR REACTION AND GOVERNING POINTS

Nogier describes three tissue layers which he calls superficial tissue, middle tissue and deep tissue. Nogier doesn't intend this concept to describe tissue in the anatomical sense, but rather it describes the ACR reaction to light touch, medium pressure (60 grams per square centimetre) and heavy pressure (110 grams per square centimetre) when applied to the skin anywhere. For practical purposes pressure can be applied by using the springloaded pressure palpator with black plastic fittings. The pressure palpator has a spring, which when fully depressed exerts a pressure of approximately 110 grams per square centimetre.

In a normal healthy person touching the skin produces no ACR reaction, but in a patient with allergic problems an ACR is often produced by simply touching the skin. If the pressure palpator is depressed halfway (exerting approximately 60 grams per square centimetre pressure) then the ACR produces a rhythmical alternation from four positive ACRs followed by four negative ACRs, followed

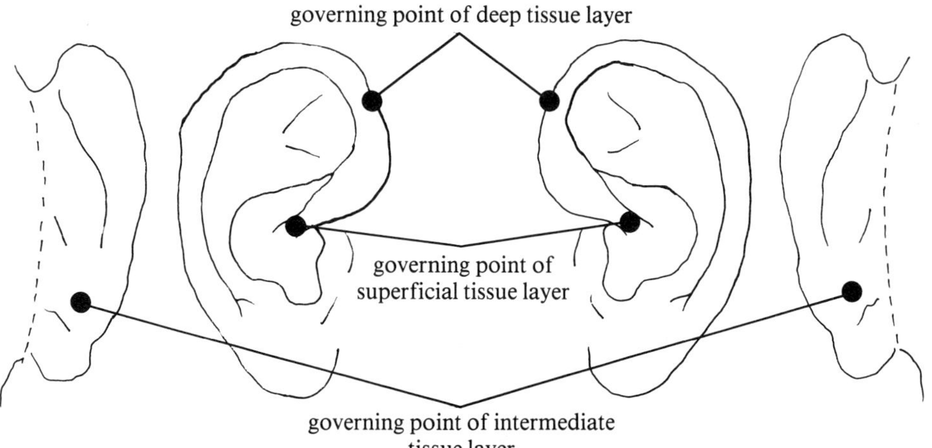

Figure 79. Governing points of the three tissue layers.

again by four positive ACRs and so on. This is regarded as a normal middle tissue reaction.

Lastly, deep pressure will produce four to eight positive ACRs followed by approximately fifteen negative ACRs; again followed by the same cycle, i.e. four to eight positive ACRs followed by fifteen negative ACRs. This is regarded as the normal deep tissue reaction.

The concept of three tissue layers ties in with the most recent concept within auricular medicine of three phases on the ear, each phase having a different position of the homunculus on the auricle (see Chapter 21). It is mentioned here to indicate the relevance of the different ACR reactions to different pressures applied to the skin. In a practical situation the ACR reaction to different pressure is of importance when examining scars. This will be described in the chapter on Toxic Scars (Chapter 16).

Governing Points of the Three Tissue Layers

Each tissue layer has a governing point, they are located at the sites shown in Figure 79. Their relevance is limited to their usefulness in determining whether inversion is present or not. Inversion is understood, in terms of auricular medicine, as being a situation in which parasympathetic areas react as if they were sympathetic, and sympathetic areas react as if they were parasympathetic. This will give 100 per cent wrong answers, and therefore ineffective treatment so it is an important situation to be aware of. It is less common than laterality instability (a relatively common) problem, especially in complex and long standing illness with pain as a presenting feature).

In a normal situation the deep tissue governing point should produce a positive ACR when a Noradrenaline ampoule is passed over it on the dominant ear; the intermediate tissue governing point should give a positive ACR when an ampoule of Acetylcholine is passed over it on the dominant side. On the dominant side the superficial tissue governing points should not be detectable at all but should only be detectable to a Noradrenaline ampoule on the non-dominant side. If these physical signs are not obtained this means that inversion is present and this has to be corrected. This can be done by needling the point of the first rib using silver, and adding a gold needle on the helix at the extremity of the radius drawn from point zero through the point of the first rib. The most efficient way, however, of correcting inversion is to apply an alternating magnetic field (alternating North/South, South/North, North/South, and so on) across the cranium; applying the poles of an electro-magnet opposite each ear for approximately three minutes. This can be done using the *Theramagnetic*.* The use of the *Theramagnetic* and also the *Theramagnetic-P* will be discussed in detail in Chapter 20.

Bahr[1] states that the governing point for the superficial tissue layer can be detected using a black/white hammer by putting a Kodak Wratten filter 44A on sympathetic skin; the intermediate tissue layer governing point by placing Kodak Wratten filter 64 on sympathetic skin, and that the deep tissue governing point can be detected using a black/white hammer by placing Kodak Wratten filter 24 on sympathetic skin. The use of these filters in the author's view is unnecessary as all three governing

Theramagnetic; available with poles situated either in headphones or on a extendable frame. The *Theramagnetic-P* is supplied with cross polaroids movable through 360° placed over each pole. Manufactured by Sedatelec.

points are detectable using Noradrenaline (deep and superficial tissue governing points) or Acetylcholine (middle tissue, or sometimes called intermediate tissue governing point). The choice of these particular three filters is not in full agreement with the three filters corresponding to each phase of the ear (see Chapter 21). This is another example of confused teaching within the school of auricular medicine, and therefore the author advises that not much importance should be attached to the use of colour filters for detecting governing points using the black/white hammer, as indicated above.

CHAPTER FOURTEEN

PROTOCOL FOR APPROACHING A PATIENT USING AURICULAR MEDICINE

The information given in the previous two chapters is summarized in the following protocol. The practitioner is recommended to follow this protocol step-by-step when using auricular medicine. The protocol refers to all the concepts and procedures detailed in the previous chapters, and therefore underlines their importance.

1. Ground the patient, using copper tube if the clinical situation so demands (i.e. when treating a patient near to X-ray apparatus or any other potential electromagnetic interference).
2. Obtain the ACR.
3. Check for laterality instability. If this is present correct this either using needles or manipulation at C7/T1.
4. Check for inversion using Noradrenaline and Acetylcholine ampoules. If inversion is present correct this, perferably using the *Theramagnetic*, or failing this using needles as for correction of laterality.
5. Place the appropriate filter on sympathetic skin. The seven colour programme is to be regarded as a general filter. Depending on the clinical situation a different filter may be selected such as a drug filter.
6. Detect pathological points, either on the dominant side alone if a non-painful condition is being treated, or if a painful condition is being treated choose the ear on the side of the pain. If the pain is midline then choose the dominant ear. Mark the pathological point(s) with a felt tip pen.
7. If point detection has been carried out using methods which do not indicate whether a gold or silver needle should be used (i.e. when point detection has been carried out using Noradrenaline in an ampoule), then determine the sort of needle, or which magnetic pole needs to be applied, using an appropriate hammer, remembering the following:

BLACK, POSITIVE AND NORTH POLE = A GOLD NEEDLE

WHITE, NEGATIVE AND SOUTH POLE = A SILVER NEEDLE

8. Having marked the pathological point with a felt tip pen record the site and needle type used on an ear diagram in the patient's notes.*
   The following symbols are recommended:

   ● = silver   ○ = gold   Δ = semi-permanent   × = steel

9. When using needles check that the needles are in the correct site using a positive/negative hammer touched against the handle of the needles.
10. Having removed the needle, or having completed treatment with a laser or with a magnetic pole, check that the point is no longer detectable.

   IF A POINT HAS BEEN ADEQUATLEY TREATED IT SHOULD NO LONGER BE DETECTABLE ON THE ACR. IF IT IS DETECTABLE, OR IF THE POINT RETURNS WITHIN MINUTES OF TREATMENT THEN FURTHER TREATMENT SHOULD BE CARRIED OUT.

11. Remove needles after they have been in place in the correct position for a sufficient period of time.

*Rubber ear stamps manufactured by Sedatelec.

CHAPTER FIFTEEN

POLAROIDS AND THEIR USE IN ACUPUNCTURE

The use of polaroids in acupuncture in general, and in auricular medicine in particular is a discovery of Nogier. The application of polaroid filters to magnets represents an interesting and useful further method of dealing with pathological points which will be discussed in detail in a later chapter.

In order to explain the ACR reaction when a polaroid is passed over the body Nogier proposes that the body has lines of force running in a longitudinal direction, rather like lines of force around a magnet. This idea is in keeping with traditional Chinese concepts in that all the meridians run in a longitudinal direction. Similar ideas have been proposed by Becker.[1,2,3] If these longitudinal lines of force are 'cut' at right angles by passing a polaroid filter with the lines of the polaroid running at right angles to the long axis of the body (see Figure 80), and if the ACR is palpated at the same time as the polaroid is passed over the skin a positive ACR is noted at certain points. These areas correspond to acupuncture points and this can be a useful method for locating areas that need to be needled; for example around a painful joint.

In very sensitive patients, that is those patients who obtain needling sensation quickly following needle insertion when using classical acupuncture, needling sensation can be obtained by simply moving the polaroid backwards and forwards, just above the skin, over an area which produces a positive ACR when polaroid is passed over it. As this sensation is produced the initially positive ACR disappears.

Therefore, a piece of polaroid can be used as a point detector, by passing the polaroid along the longitudinal axis of the body, with the lines of the polaroid running at right angles to this long axis, as indicated in Figure 80. A polaroid point detector can be made by cutting a small circle of polaroid and inserting it into the end of a pencil (Figure 81).

The German school of auricular medicine has claimed that using the polaroid as a point detector and noting when a positive ACR is obtained over particular areas of the body, that all such points so detected are 'biologically active' and should be treated. In the author's experience this is not correct as all the more useful, and therefore commonly used, classical acupuncture points are nearly always detected, such as Ho Ku (LI4), Tsu San Li (Stomach 36) etc. The polaroid comes into its own in detecting spinal levels which need needling in the case of pain originating in the spinal column, or for determining which points need to be needled around a painful

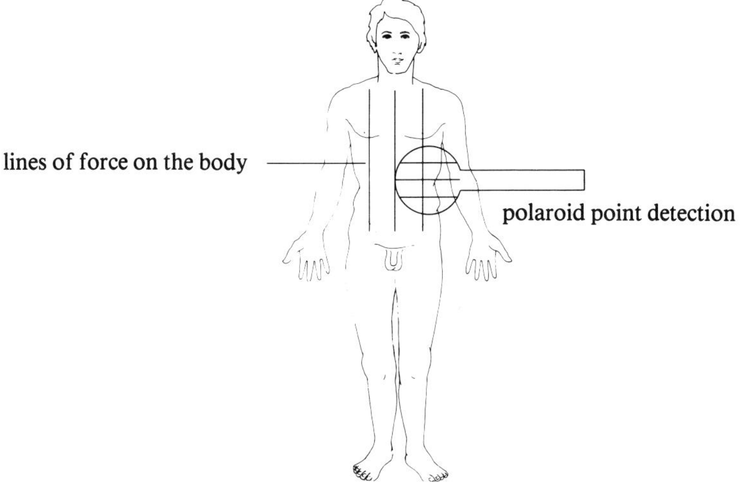

Figure 80. Diagram showing lines of force on the body being 'cut' by a polaroid with lines running at right angles to these lines.

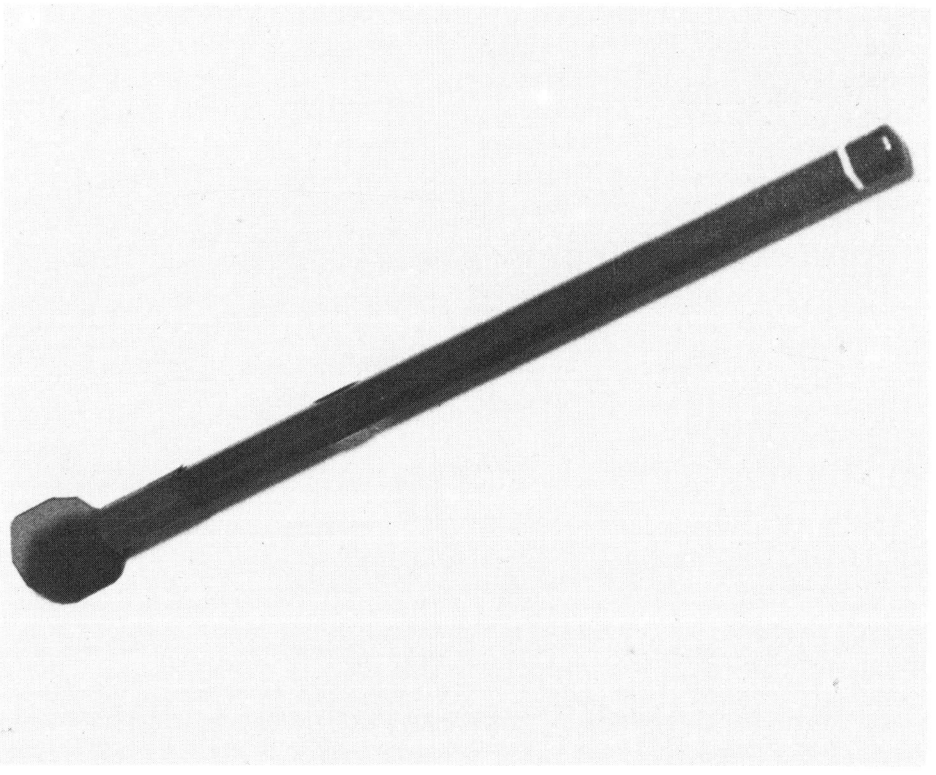

Figure 81. Polaroid point detector.

joint. In classical acupuncture practice methods for detecting these points amount to deep palpation around the joint looking for tender areas. The polaroid point detector provides a more accurate method of locating these points.

As well as the use of polaroids for point detection Nogier teaches that the orientation of the longitudinal lines of energy running up and down the body can be studied in a direct fashion, by placing a square of polaroid on the patient's forehead with the lines of the polaroid running in the longitudinal direction, i.e. from top to bottom. On rotation of the lower edge of this polaroid square, away from the midline, either to the right or to the left, at an angle of between 10 to 15 degrees from the midline a positive ACR will be noted. This is taken as indicating

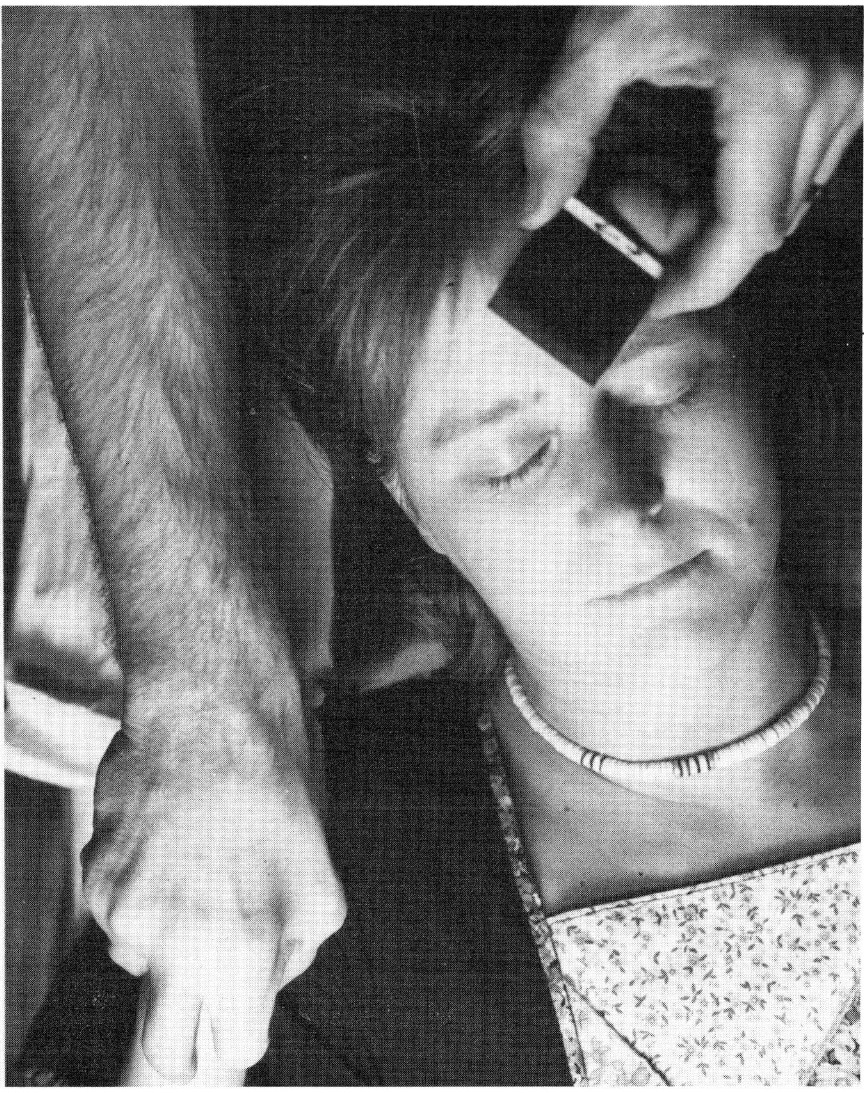

Figure 81a. Measuring the angle from the midline at which a rotating polaroid produces a positive ACR.

that the patient's energy lines are in the right orientation. The evidence for this assumption is that this is found to be a normal reaction. In illness, then the angle when a positive ACR is obtained on rotating the polaroid away from the midline is more than the normal of approximately 10 to 15 degrees. The greater the angle then, generally speaking, the iller the patient is. This provides a useful means of assessing the efficacy of therapy; in other words, if the angle from the midline is measured prior to treatment using the polaroid square, as illustrated in Figure 81a and this measurement is repeated after therapy, then if the angle has decreased therapy can be taken as having been useful. The closer that the angle at which a positive ACR occurs can be brought to normal then the more effective can the therapy be adjudged to have been. This method of testing is useful when assessing a choice of homoeopathic remedy and this will be discussed in Chapter 17. The normal angle of the energy lines from the midline of approximately 10 to 15 degrees may well have some relationship with the angle of the earth's magnetic axis to the vertical. As will become apparent later the relationship of magnetism with reference to the body's energy lines seems particularly relevant.

No plausible explanation has yet been given as to why polaroids should produce this effect, but it remains a simple and useful method of point detection. Its aplication to therapy can be either by creating needling sensation using a polaroid on the patient, as indicated above, or applying crossed polaroids over magnets (this will be described later). It is interesting to note that in polaroid sunglasses the lines of the polaroid run vertically. If the polaroid is arranged so that the lines run horizontally wearers often report headaches. This is an observed fact for which, as yet, no explanation is available. This does not apply when circular polaroid is used (where the lines are arranged in concentric circles). This sort of polaroid is useless for point detection and longitudinal polaroid, i.e. with parallel lines, is the polaroid to use.

CHAPTER SIXTEEN

POLAROIDS AND THEIR USE IN TOXIC SCARS (NEURAL THERAPY)

During the 1920s a German doctor, Dr Ferdinand Huneke, discovered that he could cure a number of cases of headache by injecting, with local anaesthetic, distant scars on the patient's body. The solution he used was Procaine Hydrochloride. Later Caffeine was added. Huneke's brother Walter Huneke, who was a dentist, together with Huneke himself repeatedly injected Procaine/Caffeine solutions into themselves in order to ascertain whether any harmful side effects could be produced.

They concluded that injection of a mixture of Procaine and Caffeine into scars had no harmful side effects, and the pharmaceutical company Bayer began to manufacture the solution under the trade name of *Impletol*.*

The Huneke brothers published their first paper in 1928 outlining this discovery and gave birth to so-called neural therapy. A number of textbooks are available on this subject,[1,2,3] all of them in German. Neural therapy has enjoyed something of a vogue in Germany, particularly amongst those doctors who practise acupuncture. Its use has not spread to any significant extent outside Germany.

At its simplest, neural therapy involves injecting all scars on a patient, including tonsillar scars, with *Impletol* in the hope of curing an apparently unrelated complaint. The fact that the scar bears no neurological relationship, nor even a relationship according to the meridians with the patient's complaint, does not appear to deter the enthusiastic neural therapist, who continues to inject all visible scars.

The injection of *Impletol* into acupuncture points is also a common practice in Germany. Unfortunately the results from neural therapy tend to be haphazard; in some cases they are excellent, and in others no results are obtained. The problem from a diagnostic point of view is for the neural therapist to decide prior to injecting scars, as to whether in the first place injecting these scars is likely to have any affect on the patient's illness, and in the second place if the answer is in the affirmative then as to which scars, or which parts of which scars need to be injected.

EAV offers a method of determining this, and this has been described in detail

Impletol is available in 2ml ampoules. Manufactured by Bayer, Leverkusen, West Germany. It is not available in the United Kingdom.

in the section on EAV in Volume I. A simpler and quicker method is available for determining if a scar is abnormal, and which parts of the scar need treatment. Therefore therapy can be specific, and only those parts of a scar yielding abnormal physical signs need be treated. In the author's experience injecting a scar along its entire length may in some cases produce results, but it often does not. However, if only those parts of the scar which produce abnormal physical signs are injected, then a higher proportion of patients gain therapeutic benefit.

Scar Examination A scar can be examined by use of a polaroid point detector and pressure palpator. A normal healthy scar will give no ACR reaction if a polaroid is passed over it, taking care to maintain the lines of the polaroid at right angles to the long axis of the body. Therefore, if a midline scar is being examined the polaroid needs to be moved down the body whilst feeling the patient's ACR (Figure 82).

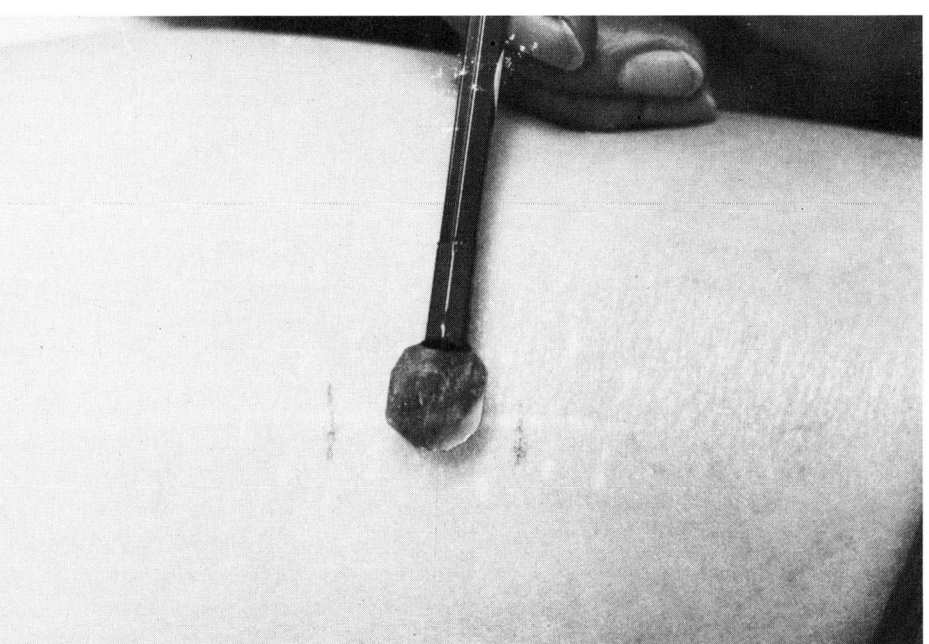

Figure 82.   Scar examination on a vertical scar (this is in the same orientation as a midline scar) using a polaroid point detector.

If a transverse scar is being examined then the polaroid should be moved from side to side, using the handle of the point detector at right angles to the long axis of the patient's body (Figure 83). If the scar is abnormal, then on passing the polaroid over the scar whilst feeling the ACR, a positive ACR will be noted over the abnormal parts of the scar. It is rare to find a scar showing this physical sign along its whole length, as generally a number of areas on a scar are found to produce this physical sign, and the change from positive ACR to a normal pulse is often marked. The appearance of the scar is no guide as to whether it is abnormal or not. This sign is as likely to be picked up on white, flat, inactive, looking scars as it is on red and angry looking scars.

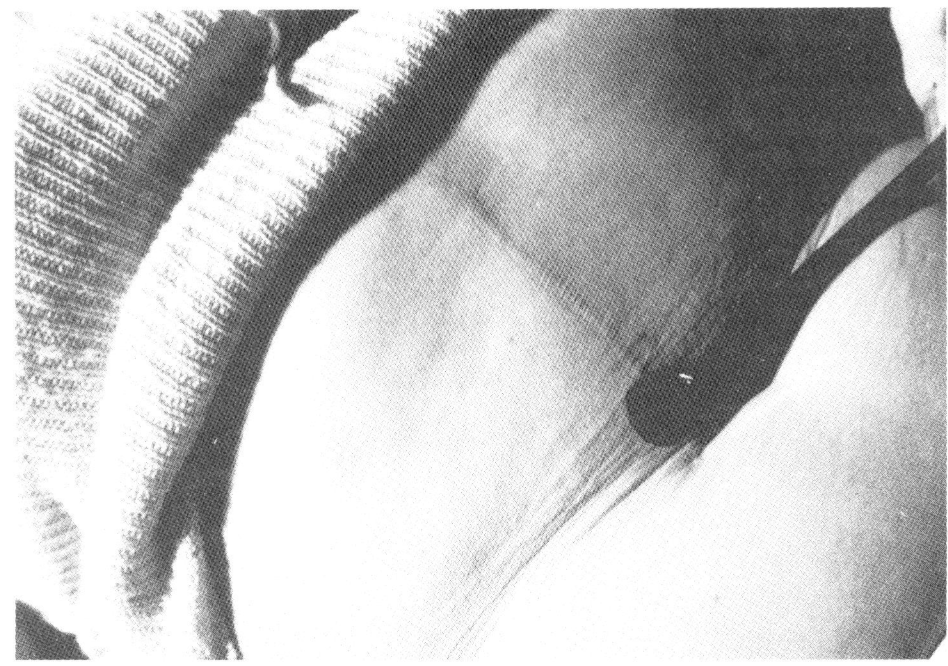

Figure 83.   Scar examination on a transverse scar using a polaroid point detector.

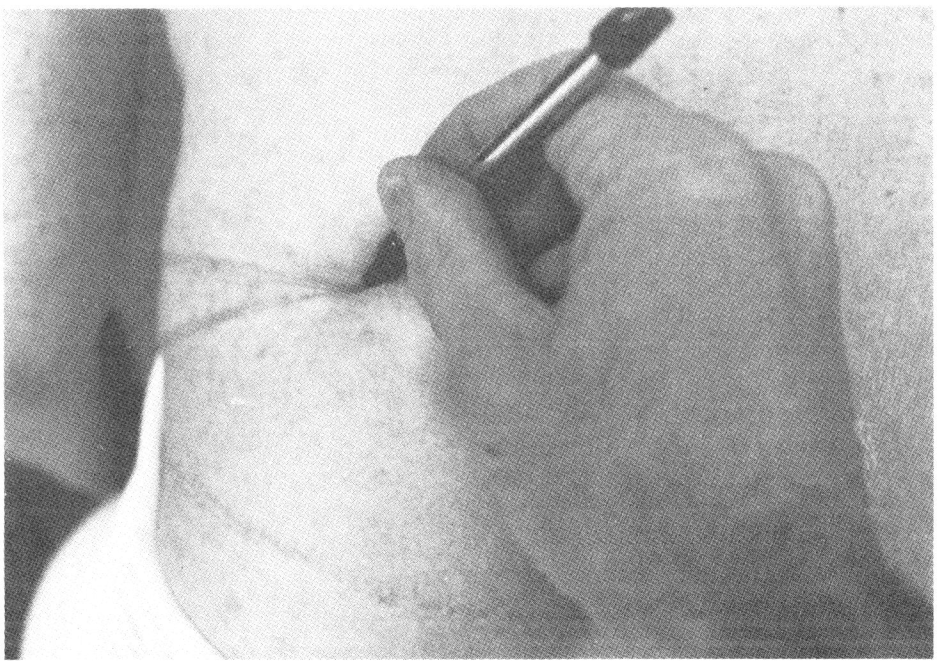

Figure 84.   Testing for a normal deep tissue reaction over a scar using the pressure palpator.

On passing the polaroid over the scar the abnormal parts of the scar should be marked, at each end of the abnormal section, with a felt tip pen.

The next step is to examine the scar with a pressure palpator. If the scar is acutely tender this can be uncomfortable for the patient and therefore reliance on the polaroid and the physical signs thereby obtained should be made. If the scar is not tender, which is often the case with scars which are successfully injected, then the pressure palpator can be used as well as the polaroid to examine the scar.

If depressed fully, whilst palpating the ACR on each section of the scar (see Figure 84) a normal scar will produce a normal deep tissue reaction; that is four to eight positive ACRs followed by approximately fifteen negative ACRs. On any abnormal part of a scar the ACR often becomes immediately negative; indeed quite markedly so in most cases. Occasionally, one, or at the most two, positive ACRs may be produced initially. Any part of any scar which shows a positive ACR on passing a polaroid over it will always show markedly negative ACRs when the pressure palpator is used over the same part of the scar. If these two physical signs are not found then the scar ought to be re-examined.

Scar Treatment *Impletol* should be drawn up into a small syringe and injected into the scar itself. This should raise a small white bleb over the scar. Injecting *Impletol* beneath the scar should be avoided, not because it is harmful, but because it will not produce any beneficial effect. Normal sterile procedure should be observed. Neural therapy, like acupuncture, requires a series of treatments. If the patient has gained some benefit from scar injection and if, on returning, the physical signs are found to be the same, i.e. positive ACR to polaroid and negative ACR to pressure palpator over the abnormal parts of the scar, then the scar should be re-injected until the physical signs become normal. This may take five or six weekly injections. The response to neural therapy is exactly the same as that for classical acupuncture, in that a proportion of patients may become temporarily worse after the first injection. Generally this doesn't occur after subsequent injections.

Small amounts only of *Impletol* are required, and no additional benefit is gained through injecting large amounts. Procaine or any other local anaesthetic may be used instead of *Impletol*.

Protocol for Scar Examination and Treatment Using Neural Therapy

1. Decide whether scars on the patient's body are likely to be important in relationship to the patient's condition, this is particularly likely to be so for example in post-laminectomy pain and in any post-operative pain situation.
2. Feel the ACR and pass the polaroid filter over all the scars on the patient's body, including scars distant and seemingly insignificant, no matter how small or inactive the scar may appear.
3. Mark the abnormal parts of any scar detected; that is those parts which yield a positive ACR when a polaroid is passed over them.
4. Check the findings made with a polaroid using the pressure palpator. This should only be used on scars which are not acutely tender. 100 per cent agreement between negative ACRs on depressing the pressure palpator over abnormal parts of any scar should be obtained as corroborative evidence.
5. Observe normal sterile procedure and inject small amounts of *Impletol* into

the scar tissue over the abnormal parts of the scar. Do not inject normal parts of scars.

6. Repeat this procedure on subsequent appointments until the abnormal physical signs (positive ACR to polaroid filters; negative ACR to pressure palpator) disappear.

7. If no clinical improvement is obtained from injecting abnormal parts of any scar detected as indicated above, after two separate attempts using neural therapy, then neural therapy should be given up as a method of treatment.

On the ear scars on other parts of the body are best treated using semi-permanent needles.

Conclusion

Neural therapy is a useful therapeutic procedure, and if the diagnostic methods outlined above are used it is possible to be specific with one's results, and not to inject *Impletol* in scars which don't require injecting. This is often what happens with practitioners using neural therapy without any diagnostic technique for assessing the normality or otherwise of any scar.

CHAPTER SEVENTEEN

THE USE OF THE ACR IN CLINICAL ECOLOGY AND HOMOEOPATHY

This chapter describes a diagnostic method developed by the author as a means of testing for food sensitivities, using the ACR as an indicator as to whether the patient is sensitive or not. As no reliable clinical or laboratory testing method has been available within the field of clinical ecology this method represents a considerable advance.

Clinical ecology refers to the area of medicine concerning disease due to environmental allergens. These may be either foods and or chemicals. Foods are the more important components of this group. Chemical sensitivities such as to hydrocarbons are not as common. When they are present they are more troublesome to deal with than food sensitivities. Clinical ecology does not refer to food allergy but more correctly calls the phenomenon a sensitivity, the reason being that serological factors accompanying conventional allergy, as in allergies to pollens, dusts etc., are often not present in food and chemical sensitivity. This has held back the progress of clinical ecology and consequently the concept of environmental disease remains a novel idea. The phenomenon of food and chemical sensitivity is poorly understood, but clinically it is useful. In many ways it falls into the same category as acupuncture in that both therapeutic methods are effective and side effect free, but both lack credibility as the explanation underlying their mode of action remains shrouded in mystery.

Clinical ecologists explain food and chemical sensitivity in terms of masked allergy. In conventional allergy, if the patient comes across the allergen an immediate reaction of some sort occurs, this is generally agreed to be immunoglobulin E (IgE) mediated. In the case of food and chemical sensitivity if the patient comes into contact with the food or chemical to which he is sensitive, initially he may notice no effect, or even get a 'lift'. Food sensitivity seems to be similar to addiction in that the patient 'feels good' initially after the 'culprit' food. Only some hours after taking the food do symptoms appear. If the patient avoids the suspect food or chemical for a period of five days and then comes into contact with this substance again, an obvious allergic-type reaction occurs and the patient immediately notices some worsening.

Ecologists claim that most of clinically important sensitivity occurs in this masked form. The fact that masked allergy does not have the same serological accompaniments in many cases, as does conventional allergy means that the term masked sensitivity is probably a more correct appellation, and the same factors make them difficult to detect. This is why a testing method useful in a clinical situation represents a considerable step forward. The author, and colleagues to whom the author has taught the method, consider that ACR detection of food and chemical sensitivities is a clinically useful method for detecting these sensitivities.

Various estimates are given as to the incidence of ecological disease depending on which author is consulted. Unfortunately the estimates differ widely, and their only common feature is that all agree that ecological disease is increasing alarmingly. In the author's practice 40per cent of patients attending have a clinically significant ecological factor in their illness. This should be taken to mean that in patients in whom ecological factors are clinically significant, avoiding substances to which they are sensitive causes an improvement, then on subsequent contact with any of these substances, the patient worsens to a greater or a lesser extent. This depends more on the frequency of re-exposure than on the amount contacted at each re-exposure.

The Incidence of Ecological Disease

Psychiatric Disease
    Depression, including some cases of manic depressive psychosis
    Anxiety
    Behaviour disorders
    Some cases of epilepsy
    Agoraphobia

ENT Disease
    Perennial rhinitis
    Chronic Sinusitis
    Glue Ear
    Recurrent Pharyngitis

Gastroenterology
    Peptic ulceration
    Coeliac disease
    Ulcerative colitis
    Crohn's disease

Skin Diseases
    Eczema
    Urticaria

Other Diseases
    Hay fever
    Asthma
    Rheumatoid arthritis

Enuresis
Migraine
General debility

More comprehensive lists are given in ecology textbooks, of which the book by
Rinkel, Randolph and Zeller[1] is recommended. In the author's experience all of
the above diseases have responded, in some cases partially, and in other cases
completely, when substances to which the patient is sensitive are avoided.

History is important in ecology and factors in the history may raise the clinician's
index of suspicion that the patient's disease is either wholly or in part ecological.
The following list of symptoms is used by the author, and if any three or more of
the following symptoms are present, then a diagnosis of food sensitivity is a real
possibility.

Each symptom need not be present all the time, and characteristically each
symptom tends to fluctuate:

1.   Persistent fatigue, not helped by rest.
2.   Over or under weight, or a history of fluctuating weight.
3.   Occasional puffiness of the face, hands, abdomen and ankles.
4.   Palpitations, particularly after food.
5.   Excessive sweating unrelated to exercise.
6.   General debility.
7.   Any symptom, the severity of which increases from morning till night. This
     increase in severity of symptoms applies to all of the above listed symptoms.

Methods of Diagnosis in Clinical Ecology The most commonly used method for the diagnosis of food allergy is fasting the
patient completely, with spring water only to drink, for a period of between seven
to fourteen days. Some practitioners allow a diet of boiled lamb and pears during
the time of the fast on the assumption that sensitivity to pears and lamb are
uncommon. This is then followed by the daily introduction of each food the patient
commonly eats, starting with the most commonly eaten food, and noting if there
is a return of symptoms.

If symptoms do not abate or disappear entirely after the fifth day of fasting then
this is taken as reliable indication the illness is not ecological. Elimination dieting
has a number of disadvantages, the most troublesome of which is the degree to
which patient co-operation is necessary and, in turn, can be obtained. In practice
this is not easy as not many patients are motivated enough to fast for the necessary
period of time. Another is that complaints related to ecological disease are often
vague, and it can be difficult for the patient to recognize any change in his condition.
This is contrary to the impression given in standard ecology texts, which leave the
reader with the impression that the results from elimination dieting are clear cut.
In the author's experience this is far from the truth. However, elimination diets
do constitute a useful method for detecting food sensitivities. The last major
disadvantage is that in most ecological disease the patient has a number of
sensitivities. If for example the patient is sensitive to three foods, then withdrawal
of one food alone may not produce alleviation of symptoms, or perhaps even the
withdrawal of two foods together may again have no effect. If all three foods are

withdrawn at the same time then the patient notices a clinical response. Therefore the right combination of foods has to be withdrawn.

In theory elimination diets should be able to recognize which combination of food is responsible. In practice, once one food has been indicted the chances of recognizing further suspect foods tends to diminish, and therefore the determination of the correct combination of foods responsible for the patient's illness is a difficult and time consuming process. Elimination dieting and introduction of foods can take anything up to six weeks to complete reliably.

In skin testing with serially diluted foods, each food concentrate, diluted by a factor of five in a base of phenol/saline (or normal saline if concentrates are stored in deep freeze) in a series of ten dilutions, is injected intradermally and the degree of whealing is taken as an indicator as to whether sensitivity to that particular food or chemical is present. This method is more reliable than elimination dieting. It also allows the selection of the correct food dilution to be given to the patient as desensitizing drops in order to 'switch off' his reaction to the food or chemical involved. The disadvantage is that it is time consuming. It can take as long as one hour to determine sensitivity to one food, and also to ascertain the dilution which the patient will need as desensitizing drops.

A number of blood tests are available; the most common is the RAST test.* RAST stands for Radio Allergo Sorbent Test. This is a test for immunoglobulin E (IgE). IgE antibodies become fixed to the surface of circulating basophils and mast cells which are tissue bound. During subsequent allergen exposure the allergen is bound by the IgE antibodies on these sensitized cells and this triggers off degranulation of histamine granules which then produces clinical symptoms. If IgE antibodies are fixed to mast cells the illness depends on the site of the mast cells involved, i.e. if they are in the joint synovium then a rheumatoid-like syndrome may develop. Similarly, if they are fixed in the bowl mucosa a colitis may develop. If these antibodies are fixed to circulating cells (basophils) then on exposure to the allergen a more generalized reaction will occur such as a widespread rash. For this test paper discs impregnated with specific anti-IgE are used. This is radioactively labelled and passed through an appropriate counter, and the presence of allergen-specific IgE is then determined.

The disadvantage of the RAST Test is that it assumes that food and chemical sensitivity is IgE mediated. There is considerable evidence to suggest that this is not so, and clearly the RAST Test is very much conceived in terms of conventional allergy. As indicated previously, much of ecology is not explicable in terms of conventional allergy. It is highly probable that at least some ecological disease is IgG and IgM mediated, or even cell mediated.

*RAST Test — Pharmacia (Great Britain) Ltd., Hounslow, Middlesex, UK.

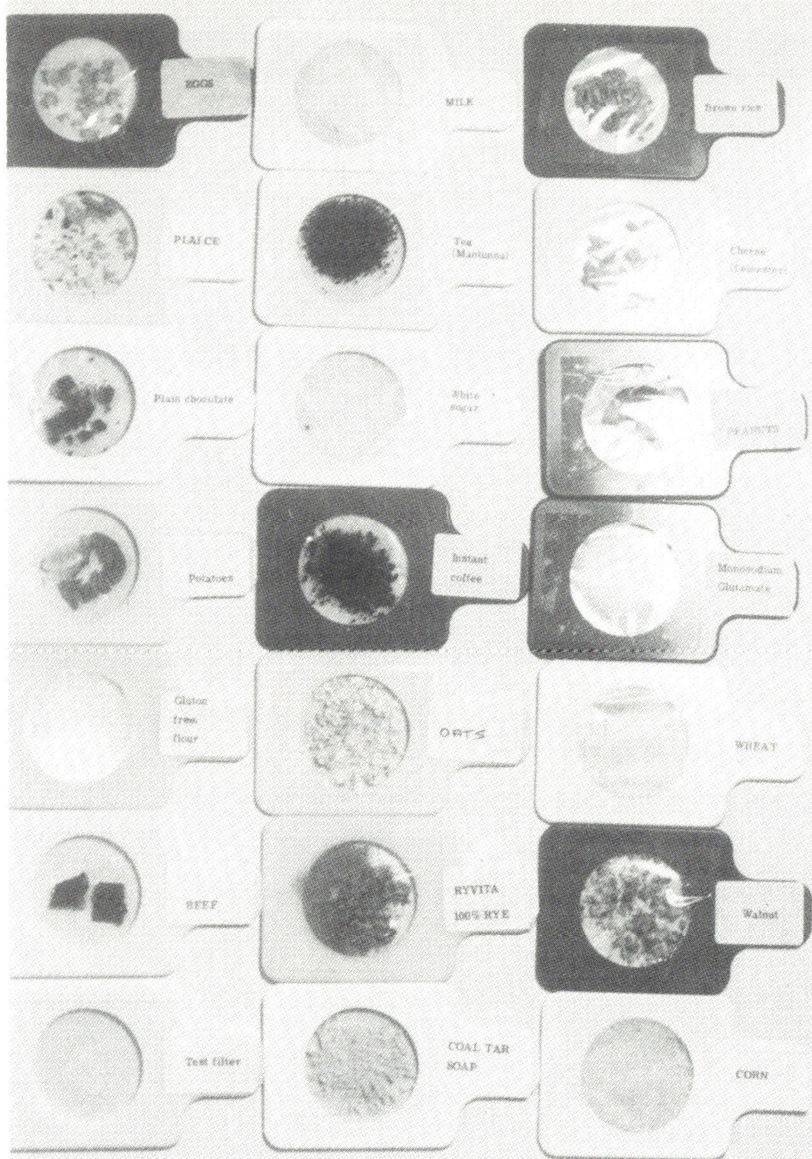

Figure 87.   Food sensitivity testing kit.

Unfortunately as a smaller area of the substances is available through which light can pass these do not give as clear a reaction on the ACR as do the filters illustrated. A blank filter is included in the set as occasionally patients are sensitive to the plastic which forms the main body of the filter. In these cases the basic testing kit cannot be used and has to be substituted by an equivalent test set made from glass serum bottles in which foods and chemicals are placed. This set is easily made up and in many cases the patient will be willing to fill a series of glass bottles with common foods and chemicals to which he is exposed.

The list of substances included in the basic testing kit follows. The items are listed in order of incidence of sensitivity occurring in the average ecology practice:

1. Milk	16. Peanuts
2. Wheat	17. Tomatoes
3. Cheese	18. Nuts
4. Bacon	19. Potatoes
5. Eggs	20. Rice
6. Citrus fruits	21. White sugar
7. Coffee	22. Fish
8. Tea	23. Standard washing powder
9. Corn	24. Gluten-free flour
10. Plain chocolate	25. Beef
11. Oats	26. Unpurified (soft brown) sugar
12. Rye	27. Tobacco
13. Hydrocarbons (i.e. Coal Tar products)	28. Decaffinated coffee
	29. Lamb
14. Biological washing powders	30. Blank test filter
15. Food additives	

The above list is by no means complete, but it provides a useful basic testing kit. Different practitioners will find different orders of incidence of food sensitivity. For example, in a practice consisting of a mainly rice eating population, sensitivity to rice will replace sensitivity to wheat as one of the most common sensitivities.

The patient is likely to be sensitive to substances to which he is most frequently exposed, therefore it can save time if the practitioner asks the patient to make a rank order of foods consumed, and only the top ten items on the list need be tested. In practice the author tests all of the basic substances in the testing kit as indicated above. The patient is then instructed on avoidance of substances to which he is found sensitive and is asked to indicate any other commonly eaten foods or commonly contacted chemicals which are not present on the list of foods tested on the first appointment, so that these can be tested at a subsequent appointment.

Protocol for Treatment of Patients with Food and/or Chemical Sensitivities

1. Having ascertained the foods and/or chemicals to which the patient is sensitive he should be advised on strict avoidance of these. Lists of foods containing wheat, milk and dairy products, eggs and corn are appended at the end of this chapter. Sensitivity to these foods is common and as they are present in many products, the patient must be advised on all of them so that avoidance can be effectively carried out. Complete avoidance applies only to those substances which give no ACR over parasympathetic skin and a positive ACR over sympathetic skin.

2. Substances which give equal ACR reaction over both parasympathetic and sympathetic skin should be regarded as equivocal. If the patient is highly allergic, and in practice this means a patient with a large number of foods and/or chemicals to which he is sensitive (i.e. more than six substances), then the foods which are giving an equivocal reaction should also be avoided.

3. In patients who are sensitive to less than six substances, the substances which have produced an equivocal reaction should at most only be taken once every third day.
4. If the patient is sensitive to six or more substances he should be instructed to rotate the diet. This means not to have any food more than once in three days. In practice this can be difficult, but it is possible and well repays the effort made.
5. If a patient is found to be sensitive to hydrocarbons, and as these are impossible to avoid (i.e. exposure to exhaust fumes), desensitization with dilutions of phenol or ethanol or dilutions of exhaust fumes bubbled through normal saline should be given.
6. Patients with large numbers of food sensitivities in which avoidance is difficult, either through reasons of a large number of sensitivities, or through inconvenience, should be treated using desensitization.

Food and Chemical Desensitization

Patients may be desensitized for substances to which they react by giving a dilution of that substance, either by sublingual drops which generally have to be taken three times daily before taking the culprit food(s) or by self administered intradermal injection approximately once every three days; more often for highly sensitive and less often for less sensitive patients. A description of food desensitization using this technique is given by Miller.[?] This method is used by the author with considerable success and is the only practical way of treating highly sensitive patients, particularly if hydrocarbon sensitivities are a major feature.

The ACR may also be used to ascertain the dilution which the patient needs to be given to 'turn off' his reaction to the substance involved. This is done by testing each of the ten serial dilutions from one through to ten. Each dilution will give a positive ACR when held over sympathetic skin until the dilution is reached that will 'switch off' the patient's reaction. When this dilution is tested, instead of giving a positive ACR over sympathetic skin, which as indicated above means sensitivity to the substance, the dilution capable of switching off the reaction will no longer give a positive ACR over sympathetic skin, and instead will give either no ACR or a negative ACR over sympathetic skin, and conversely a positive ACR over parasympathetic skin.

Conclusion

The ACR is a quick and cheap clinical test for diagnosing food and chemical sensitivities. It is possible to determine which food and/or chemical the patient should avoid as well as advising which foods he is able to eat. In many ways this is more helpful than telling him which foods he cannot eat. Experience shows that it is also possible to obtain the correct desensitizing dilution using the ACR; again this is a quicker method than intradermal testing, even though intradermal testing is a reliable method.

The experience of the author when comparing results obtained using the ACR as a diagnostic method with results obtained from RAST Tests has been that often no direct correlation is obtained. This falls into line with the supposition that food and chemical sensitivity is not always an IgE mediated phenomena. In a few cases a positive correlation between RAST Tests and the ACR food and chemical test is obtained, but nearly always ACR testing produces a wider range of sensitivities, and therefore in clinical practice probably gives better and more clearcut results than other testing methods. As there is no generally accepted serological test for food and chemical sensitivity the evaluation of the ACR detection method for diagnosing these sensitivities rests on clinical grounds as does much of ecology at the present time.

In clinical practice the ACR, if competently used, can be relied upon to produce the right answers in 90 per cent of ecological illness after two separate testing sessions; the first session being devoted to a testing of the basic set of foods and chemicals, and the second devoted to checking of the first session and testing of substances present in the patient's environment but which were omitted on the first test. These clinical results can be confirmed as with standard ecology by the patient being advised to try taking the suspect foods, or coming into contact with the suspected chemicals again when a worsening of the patient's condition should be observed if the diagnosis is correct.

The Use of the ACR in Selecting Homoeopathic Medications

It will be apparent from ACR testing for sensitivities that it is not only possible to detect if a patient is sensitive to a substance but it is also possible to determine if a patient needs a substance, and this can be used to choose a homoeopathic remedy or an antibiotic or analgesic. The method used is the reverse of that used for detecting sensitivities. Firstly bottles of the range of remedies to be tested are obtained and passed from parasympathetic to sympathetic skin. If the patient requires the remedy then a positive ACR will occur over parasympathetic skin and no ACR, or perhaps a negative ACR, will occur over sympathetic skin. The use of the ACR in this situation has merits in that it is quick and simple to perform. Similarly, analgesics can be chosen for a patient, or an antibiotic can be selected, also sensitivities to

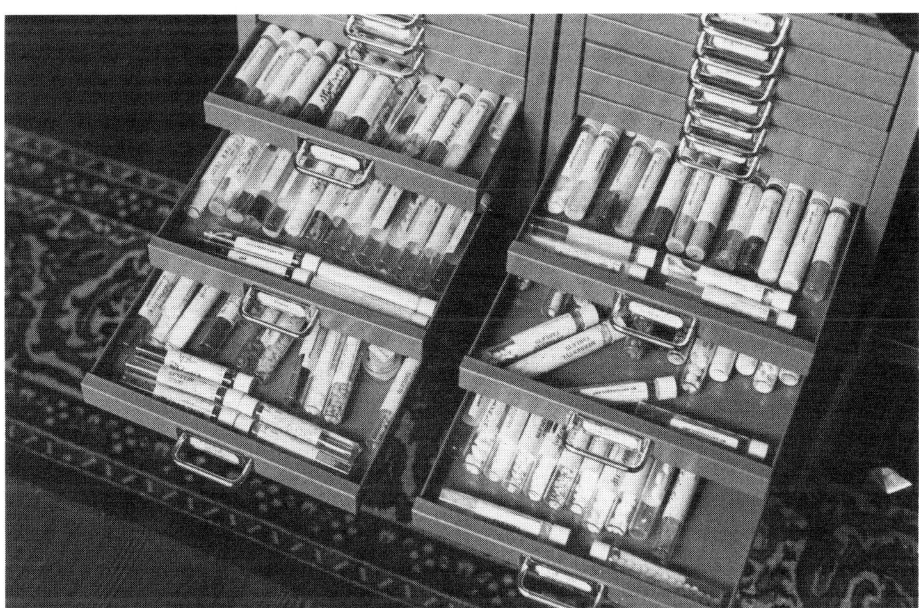

Figure 87a.   Collection of drugs and chemicals in bottles for sensitivity testing.

drugs can be detected. The author has built up a wide selection of drugs in bottles for such testing (Figure 87a).

Any drug which comes with a coating or plastic capsule should first be emptied out of its capsule, or the coating removed before putting the drug into the test bottle.

In theory it should be possible to quantify the degree to which a patient is sensitive to any substance, or indeed the degree to which a patient needs any substance; for example in the case of an antibiotic, analgesic or a homoeopathic remedy etc. This can be done by testing the number of positive ACRs occurring when a substance is held against either parasympathetic or sympathetic skin, depending on whether the substance is needed or whether it ought to be removed from the patient's environment. In practice this is difficult to detect, as it is not as easy to decide when a positive ACR becomes negative, whereas it is simpler to detect a negative ACR or a normal pulse becoming positive. Counting the number of beats for positive ACRs presupposes being able to accurately determine as to whether the ACR reverts back to normal, or to the negative state. Equipment for recording the ACR may change the situation (see Appendix at the end of this section on Electronic Recording of the ACR). A sophistication of the above described method for selection of homoeopathic remedies is to use a polaroid filter.

A Combination Method Using Polaroids and the ACR for Homoeopathic Medicine Selection

The best way of deciding which homoeopathic remedy to give the patient is to use a polaroid square placed on the patient's forehead with the lines running from top to bottom; in other words in line with the Renmo. The angle of rotation from the midline which produces a positive ACR is noted, then each homoeopathic remedy to be tested is placed in the patient's hand one by one. If a remedy is going to be useful then on retaking the ACR after placing each successive remedy in the patient's hand the angle from the midline at which a positive ACR is obtained by rotation of the polaroid will decrease.

On a number of occasions it will be noted that on placing another remedy in the patient's hand the angle will not change at all, or only slightly or even in some cases the angle will increase. These remedies can be dispensed with and only those remedies which produce a diminution of the angle to the normal (approximately ten to fifteen degrees from the vertical) should be chosen for the patient. This is a useful way of reducing the number of nosodes and accompanying remedies to be given to a patient as detected when using medicine testing in electro-acupuncture according to Voll (see Volume I, Chapter 12). This counters the tendency of medicine testing in EAV to produce too big a range of remedies. It is not uncommon for twenty to thirty remedies to be indicated using medicine testing according to EAV, and it has been pointed out in the section on medicine testing in EAV that it is not unknown to see some practitioners of EAV give sixty and above nosodes and accompanying remedies simultaneously as therapy. This is no way reflects on the validity of EAV medicine testing but rather, in the author's view, is one of the shortcomings of medicine testing using EAV. This shortcoming can be overcome by use of this simple test with a polaroid.

Summary

The information contained in the present chapter can be summarized into the following:

1. A positive ACR occurring when any substance is held over sympathetic skin indicates sensitivity to that substance.
2. A positive ACR occurring to any substance held over parasympathetic skin indicates that the patient requires that substance.

If the above is regarded as a rule of thumb then confusion is unlikely to result.

APPENDIX

Lists of foods which contain the four most commonly indicted foods responsible for much of food related ecological disease are given here.

For patients to successfully avoid these foods (as they are present in many commonly eaten dishes) the following information must be known to the patient and he should be advised to check the ingredients (listed compulsorily in Britain) on every item of packaged food:

1. *Instructions for avoidance of milk and dairy products.*

The patient should be advised to avoid the following:

Cows milk (even in very small quantities)	Dairy ice cream
	Condensed milk
Creamed foods	Dried evaporated milk
Creamed sauces	Powdered milk
Fresh cream	Malted milk
Cheeses of every description	*Ovaltine*
Custards	Salad dressings
Milk chocolate	Soups with milk added
Cakes in which milk is used	Whey
Butter	Yogurt
Foods fried in butter	

If the patient is very sensitive to milk he would be advised to use Whey-free margarine such as *Tomor* (Kosher Margarine). Unless otherwise stated milk sensitive patients are able to have Goats milk or Soya milk substitute as alternatives.

2. *If the patient is sensitive to wheat, the following foods must be avoided:*

Bread made from wheat flour, whether white or brown.

Rye flour (most rye flour contains a proportion of wheat. Only if the patient is absolutely sure that the rye flour contains no wheat can he then have rye flour).

Gluten-free flour (unless the patient is sensitive only to gluten in).

Ovaltine	*Weetabix*
Wheat cereals such as:	Grape Nuts
Puffed Wheat	All Bran
Shredded Wheat	Biscuits

Doughnuts
Pies
Sponge puddings
Suet puddings
Gravies and sauces in which wheat
    is used for thickening
Cakes (most cakes are made from
    wheat products)
Wheat germ
Sausages (most sausages contain
    wheat in the form of a cereal
    binder)

Pasta
Rusks
Dumplings
Fish fingers and other fish dishes
    coated in breadcrumbs
Batters
Semolina
Tapioca

3. *If the patient is sensitive to eggs the following foods should be avoided:*

Eggs
Cakes
Custards
Hamburgers (the meat loaf is
    mixed with egg white to give
    adhesion)
Icings
Macaroni

Malted cocoa (i.e. drinks such as
    Ovaltine etc.)
Egg noodles
Pancakes
Soufflés
Mayonnaise, salad creams
Sausages (often bound with egg)

4. *If the patient is sensitive to corn (maize) he should be advised to avoid the
following:*

Corn flakes
Corn flour
Corn meal
Corn oil i.e. *Mazola*
Corn starch
Corn syrups such as *Sweetose* or
    glucose syrup
Popcorn
Corn on the cob
Canned corn
Cough syrup
Chewing gums

Gummed papers such as on
    envelopes, labels, stamps etc.
Ice creams
Malt
Talcum powder (these often
    contain corn)
Jams (often contain glucose syrup)
Beer   } (contain malt)
Whisky
Rice Krispies (these contain corn in
    the form of malt)
Sausages (corn in the cereal binder)
Creamed soups

CHAPTER EIGHTEEN

THE BIOLOGICAL EFFECTS OF ELECTROMAGNETIC FIELDS

Before outlining the use of magnetic fields and lasers in acupuncture it is important to understand the nature of applied electromagnetic energy and something about the biological effects of electromagnetic radiation. Such effects are being studied with increasing interest, and now a vast array of carefully executed studies are available in the research literature. Most of this work has been carried out by biophysicists with, as yet, relatively little contribution from the medical profession. It is not surprising that doctors whose scientific training tends to predominate in the fields of biology and chemistry rather than of maths and physics are somewhat daunted by the seemingly unintelligible mathematical nature of many of these papers. In the author's view this information has to become accessible to clinicians working in this area of medicine, as it provides a sensible means of further investigation, combined with measurement, and also opens up possible explanations for the phenomenon of acupuncture.

Introduction

The effects of electric and magnetic energy in space is described in terms of fields, within which the electric and magnetic force acts. Electric and magnetic fields are both vectors; this means that they both have magnitude and direction. Both electric charges and magnetic poles exert forces on one another. The force (F) between two static charges (q1) and (q2) being a distance apart (d) is described by Coulomb's Law:

$$F = \frac{q1 \cdot q2}{+ d^2} \cdot k$$

where k = a constant. This is an application to electromagnetism of the inverse square law. Magnetic field strength could be substituted for charge (q) in Coulomb's law.

Any electric current, which in simple terms is a movement of charge, produces a magnetic field. Conversely, a changing magnetic field induces an electromotive

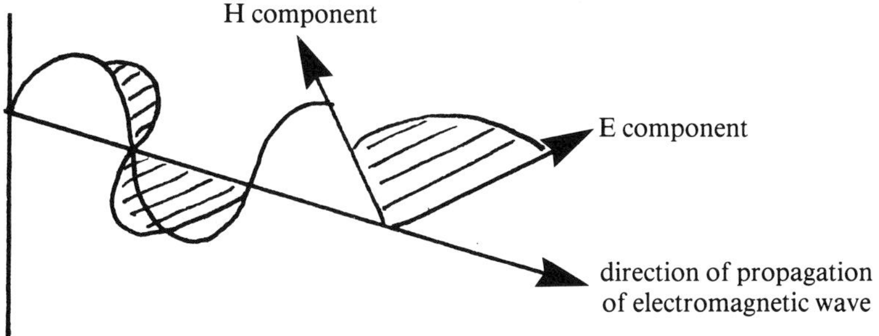

Figure 88.　　Diagram showing electric and magnetic components of an electromagnetic wave.

force. The magnitude of this induced electromotive force is proportional to the strength of the magnetic field involved, and on the rate of change of the magnetic field. Therefore a moving magnet can induce a current. This close relationship between electric and magnetic forces is of fundamental importance relative to electromagnetic waves, in that every electromagnetic wave has an electric and a magnetic component which are at right angles to each other; this is illustrated in Figure 88. By convention, the magnetic component is designated H and the electric component E.

Electromagnetic energy is transmitted in the form of waves, and these waves are systematized according to their frequency and wavelength into the electromagnetic spectrum; this is summarized in Figure 89.

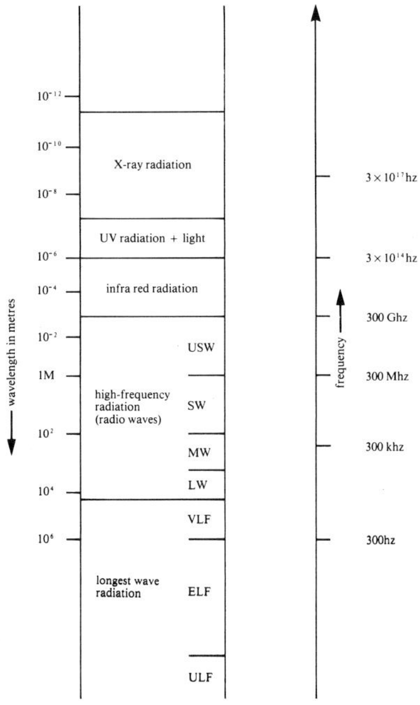

Figure 89.　　The Electromagnetic spectrum.

Biological effects of electromagnetic radiation occur firstly within the ULF (ultra low frequency), the ELF (extremely low frequency) and the VLF (very low frequency) ranges. No further significant biological effects are noted until the millimetre-centimetre wave region is reached. All electromagnetic radiations above this, going up from infra red to visible light, on to ultra violet radiation, and then finally to X-ray and cosmic radiation are all noted to have biological effects. The greater the frequency of the electromagnetic wave, and therefore by implication the greater its energy content, then the more damaging are its biological effects.

Konig[1] considers that the biological implications of electromagnetic fields provide indirect confirmation for the hypothesis that these fields have an important evolutionary role. Pressman[2] similarly concludes that enough direct and indirect evidence now exists to support the claim that electromagnetic forces in general must play a role of an as yet incalculable importance in information transfer between and within living organisms. Konig sums up the present situation as follows:

> If one starts out from the facts as presented by modern classical physics, thereby ruling out the possible existence of any mysterious, or as yet undiscovered forces or energy forms, then there must ultimately be a smooth transition between the observed processes and the theoretical model. However, this can only be fully accepted if and when there is a corresponding link between physics and physiology, also providing such a smooth transition between these two disciplines.

It is clear from reviewing the copious number of papers on the biological effects of electromagnetic fields, that as yet there is no corresponding link between physics and physiology, and many of the phenomena repeatedly observed in these investigations remain beyond scientific explanation at the present time.

Pressman[2] summarizes what the majority of researchers have found when studying the biological effects of electromagnetic fields on living organisms:

> The practical procedure when investigating the reactions of the entire organism to electromagnetic fields is then to go on from there to determine the simplest level of organization at which it is still possible to detect the changes which are ultimately responsible for the particular reaction of the organism. The prime cause of the reaction need not necessarily be due to processes at the molecular level — it may be a feature of some macroscopic level of organization. There is nothing paradoxical in this — we encounter such a situation in the examination of 'organized' machine systems, which are also characterized by the presence of a hierarchy of order, and the appearance of new properties with increasing complexity.
>
> This can be illustrated by the example of such a relatively simple system as the oscillatory circuit. The specific feature of this circuit is its particularly high sensitivity to an electromagnetic field of a particular (resonant) frequency. Of course, the electromagnetic oscillations induced in the circuit, are due to microprocesses — motion of electrons in the wires and the polarization of the molecules in the dielectric of the capacitor. But attempts to discover the mechanism of resonance at this level will be in vain — it is not there. Nor can we detect this property by considering the processes in separate microscopic elements of the circuit — the capacitor and the induction coil. The property of resonance is a feature only of the whole organized system — the circuit as a whole.
>
> Thus, the phenomenological approach to the investigation of the systems and processes involved in the reactions of biological systems to electromagnetic fields is a practical one at present.

This quotation from Pressman is clearly relevant to the system of acupuncture, which is a system that works in its complexity rather than in its individual parts. Therefore it may well be that the approach to studying the effects of acupuncture should be more in line with the approach of the biophysicists, as typified by Pressman, in their approach to the scientific study of the biological effects of electromagnetic fields.

Characteristics of Biologically Active Electromagnetic Fields The most universally agreed observation of characteristics of biologically active electromagnetic fields is that the intensity has to be very low indeed; in some cases so low that equipment able to measure such low field strengths has only recently become available. Paradoxically, if the strength of the applied electromagnetic field is increased then the organism ceases to react to the applied energy. Numerous examples are available in the literature of biological systems responding only to applied electromagnetic fields within a narrow intensity range. These intensities have nearly always been very low indeed.[1,2,3,4,5] Exposure of the head to electromagnetic fields has been uniformly found to cause greater effects than whole body exposure. Auricular medicine applies this finding in a useful way by applying electromagnetic energy to points on the ear, thereby applying electromagnetic energy to the head, and by applying magnetic fields across the cranium. The position of the long axis of the body relative to the plain of polarization of the electromagnetic wave has also been found to be relevant. In one experiment, carried out by Addington and Deichman[6,7] placing the long axis of experimental animals perpendicular to the plane of polarization of an applied electromagnetic wave resulted in none of the experimental animals being killed. However, when the animals were placed with their long axis parallel to the plain of polarization of the wave, all the animals died.

Perhaps the most characteristic feature of all biologically effective electromagnetic waves is their pulsed nature. The relevance of the frequency of pulsation of electromagnetic waves, and the phenomena of resonance has been alluded to in the quote from Pressman. This is also relevant in the application of frequencies to each of the seven zones of the ear as described by Nogier. The ACR in this situation may well be indicating the presence of a resonance effect. If a resonance effect occurs in biological systems then only minute amounts of applied energy are required in order to produce a seemingly inordinate response. This is best illustrated by the biological effects of electromagnetic waves at the lowest end of the spectrum (ULF and ELF frequencies). There are natural rhythms tuned around the basic frequency of ten cycles per second (10 hz). This corresponds to the so-called Schumann resonance[8] which occurs at approximately ten cycles per second due to the excitation of the earth-ionosphere cavity resonator by thunder storm activity. In this case the earth and the ionosphere act like a gigantic capacitor with the earth being the negative and the ionosphere the positive plate. It appears that biological organisms have harmonized themselves via resonance phenomena to this basic rhythm; this is well illustrated in its relationship to brain rhythms. Wiener[9] conducted harmonic analysis of the alpha rhythm of brain biopotentials, and expressed the hypothesis that the brain contains several generators with frequencies close to 10 hertz. These findings may explain why a frequency of stimulation of around 10 hertz is noted to have marked beneficial effects (see section

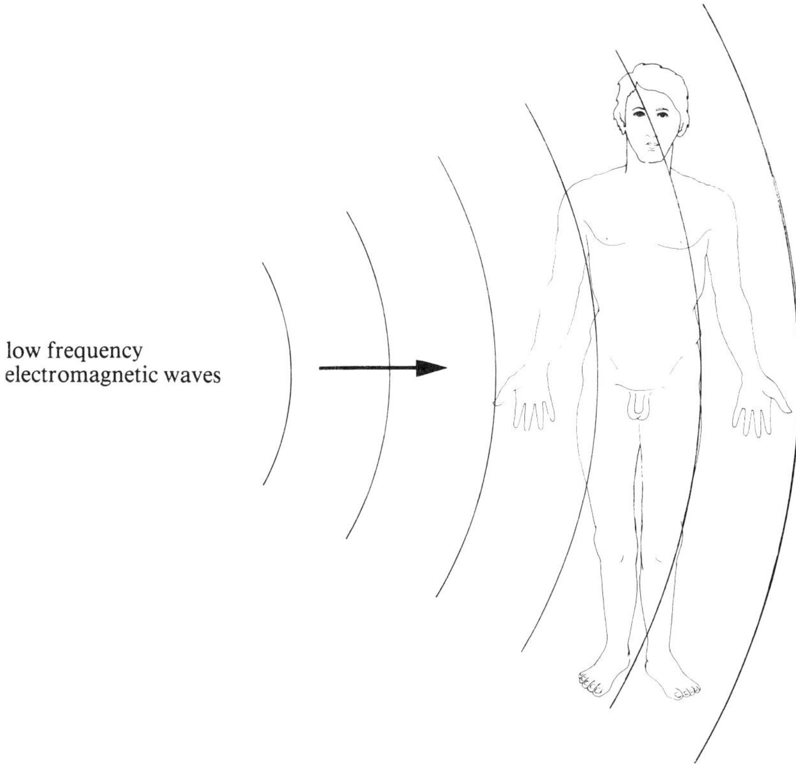

Figure 90.   Diagram illustrating that low frequency electromagnetic waves penetrate biomatter entirely.

on Neuro-electric Therapy in Volume I).

Low frequency signals such as those produced by the Schumann resonance have very long wavelengths. This means that they penetrate the entire body more or less effectively. A specific transfer of this signal to any particular place in the body is out of the question as the signal stimulus from a low frequency electromagnetic wave is present all over the body. This situation is illustrated diagramatically in Figure 90.

This therefore means that naturally occurring electromagnetic fields of low frequencies and long wavelengths (that is in the ULF, ELF, and VLF ranges) are likely to be signals to which natural biological rhythms such as circadian rhythms are synchronized, and this is indeed found to be the case. The major part of research into biological effects of electromagnetic fields has concerned this lower end of the spectrum, perhaps because a good deal is known about natural biological rhythms and also about these natural electromagnetic fields, and also it is not necessary to postulate any particular physiological receptor mechanism to explain the biological effects of these low frequency fields.

The situation is completely different when considering biological effects of high frequency electromagnetic fields such as those in the microwave region and above. These extremely short wave types of radiation propagate much more favourably

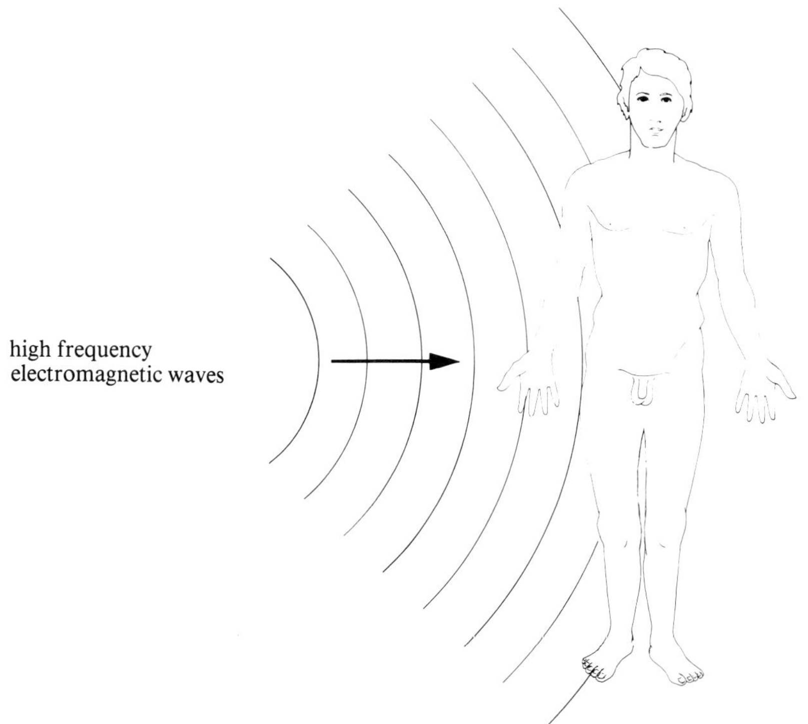

Figure 91.   Diagram illustrating that high frequency electromagnetic waves are stopped at the surface of the body.

than low frequency electromagnetic fields in that high frequency fields can be beamed, and they are also more easily absorbed by matter. They do not penetrate the body to any significant extent, as the size of the body is big in comparison to the wavelength of the applied field. This therefore means that in order for these high frequency fields to have biological effects the receiving site (the receptor) must be placed on the surface of the body, this is shown diagramatically in Figure 91.

This therefore means that high frequency radiation which includes microwave, centimetre waves, infra-red, visible light and ultra violet radiation can be aimed to a particular part of the body, but a receptor must be present on the surface of the body in order for such a field to have any biological effect. There also has to be some mechanism within the body for the transfer of this information from the receptor on the surface of the skin, so that the information contained in the field may pass to its effector site. This is where our understanding of the physiology of the biological effects of these high frequency fields breaks down, and it is in this situation where acupuncture points and the system of meridians offers a possible explanation. The most commonly noted feature of acupuncture is the existence of the acupuncture point. This feature of acupuncture was the feature recognized by the originators of traditional Chinese medicine, and around which the system has been built. This is a salient feature of Porkert's book *The Theoretical Foundations of Chinese Medicine.*[10]

Acupuncture points have been shown to lie below areas of increased skin conductivity. This has been found by a number of researchers; the most extensive studies in this area have been done by Becker[11]. Lastly, acupuncture points have been successfully rendered visible by a technique termed 'electronography', a sophisticated development of Kirlain photography. This work has been carried out by Dumitrescu[12]. As yet this work concerning the visualization of acupuncture points has not been repeated, but it is hoped that with the author's edition of a translated text of Dumitrescu's[12] describing his technique, that it may enable other researchers to repeat Dumitrescu's findings.

In conclusion, therefore, a strong biophysical case can be made for the existence of acupuncture points. The existence of meridians, however, remains an as yet unproven concept, even though in the practical situation meridians seem to 'work'.

It would appear sensible that the application of electromagnetic fields in the high frequency range could produce biological effects, and therefore be useful in acupuncture, and indeed this is what is found. The use of waves in the millimetre-centimetre waveband (microwaves) is contra-indicated as these are dangerous. It is interesting to note that the safety levels for exposure to microwaves as laid down in the United States are ten times higher than those laid down by the Soviet authorities. This area of the electromagnetic spectrum remains one of great interest, and one in which much investigation is continuing. The application of electromagnetic fields in the infra red range is the area in which applied energy to acupuncture points is most commonly used. In this case, laser radiation is applied. This will be discussed in more detail in Chapter 19.

The therapeutic application of pulsed magnetic fields is a potentially useful clinical application of magnetism. Research on this area of therapy is surprisingly limited in view of the equipment marketed by various firms for the application of pulsed magnetic fields in various clinical situations. Only one of the main texts on the biological effects of electromagnetic fields[2] mentions anything about the application of electromagnetic fields in therapy, and then this only occupies four pages of the book (pages 269-272). Most research in the therapeutic application of pulsed magnetic fields has been carried out in the field of fracture repair, particularly in fracture non-union. Most of this work has been carried out by Bassett[5] and this work has had considerable impact on orthopaedics. However, work done on the effects of pulsating magnetic fields on bone healing has come in for some justified criticism[13] in that as yet no controlled trials have been undertaken. When applying magnetic fields in therapy it is found that low frequency fields are more effective than high frequency fields, and that the findings have been exactly the same as the researchers in the field of biological effects of electromagnetic fields, in that extremely low intensity fields were required in order to produce a biological effect; increasing the strength of the applied field tending to produce a loss of therapeutic effect. When applying such low frequency fields the necessity of having a receptor on the surface of the body does not arise as these fields permeate throughout living tissue. There can be no doubt that pulsed magnetic fields have major therapeutic benefit when applied to bone; as to whether such benefits occur in other situations is not clear at the moment. These facts should be borne in mind when reading the section on the application of pulsed magnetic fields in situations other than for fracture healing (see later).

A favoured explanation of the mechanism of action of pulsating magnetic fields in therapy is that any magnetic field will produce an electric field at right angles to it within the tissues. This will in turn cause ionic movement within the tissues with the same frequency as the applied pulsed magnetic field. Above a particular frequency more rapid tonic movement is precluded by physical factors within the tissues such as ionic size and their situation, whether they be in a cell membrane or in a fluid medium. This may be one of the reasons why very low frequencies are the most biologically effective, as this ionic movement may have some ordering effect in growth and healing processes. The direction of movement of the ions will be governed by their charge. The question as to why biological systems respond to extremely weak signals remains, as the signal to noise ratio is heavily weighted in favour of noise arising from interfering signals in the environment. This therefore makes it unlikely that any receptor will pick up an ultra weak signal within such a lot of interference. One suggested possibility is that ultra weak signals, if they act for sufficient time, will be picked out by biological receptors. This problem, however, remains unexplained. When applying energy, such as lasers or magnetic energy, to acupuncture points then the ratio becomes balanced more in favour of the signal, in that the energy is supplied directly onto the acupuncture point, and therefore the effect of interfering fields in the environment is lessened. It is important to carry out such therapy in a situation as free from interference from outside electromagnetic fields as possible, such as X-ray installations, television and radio transmitters etc.

CHAPTER NINETEEN

LASERS AND THEIR USE IN AURICULAR THERAPY AND ACUPUNCTURE

Laser means light amplification by stimulated emission of radiation. This is the process that takes place inside the device. The lasers used for acupuncture and auricular therapy are semi-conductor lasers, and are low powered devices. Powers ranging from 2 to 5 milliwatts is typical of the power output of lasers used in acupuncture. The skin penetration of the laser beam is at the most 3 millimetres, this however depends on the power of laser being used, but it can be generally assumed that laser radiation from acupuncture therapy devices will not penetrate below 3 millimetres. This limits their use when classical acupuncture points are stimulated, as many classical acupuncture points lie considerably deeper beneath the skin than 3 millimetres, and in the author's opinion the use of laser therapy on classical acupuncture points is of little value unless it is specifically used on points situated close to the surface, i.e. those on hands, feet and the ear.

The use of the laser on ear points is a different matter as all points on the ear are situated close to the surface, and they may all be treated effectively by the use of laser radiation. In order to understand the application of laser radiation to acupuncture points it is important to know the principles on which the laser is based.

Basic Principles of Laser Action

The characteristics of radiation emitted from a laser are that this radiation is in phase, both in time and space. This is illustrated diagrammatically in Figure 92. This means that the emitted light is coherent. Lasers used in acupuncture use a semi-conductor as the material which is made to lase. The *Theralaser** uses gallium-arsenide as a semi-conductor. This is present in the device as a cylinder with a mirror at one end, and another mirror, but only 95 per cent reflective, at the emission end of the laser. This is illustrated diagrammatically in Figure 93.

Energy is applied to the semi-conductor which has the effect of raising the energy level of electrons present in the substance in which laser action is to be stimulated, and this is achieved by the addition of photons which can be regarded as packets

**Theralaser* manufactured by Sedatelec, 135 Route Neuve, Irigny, France.

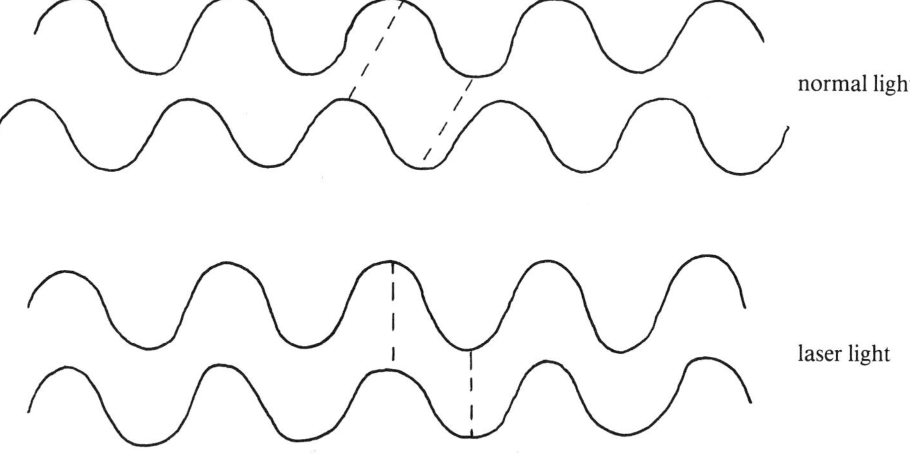

Figure 92. Laser radiation.

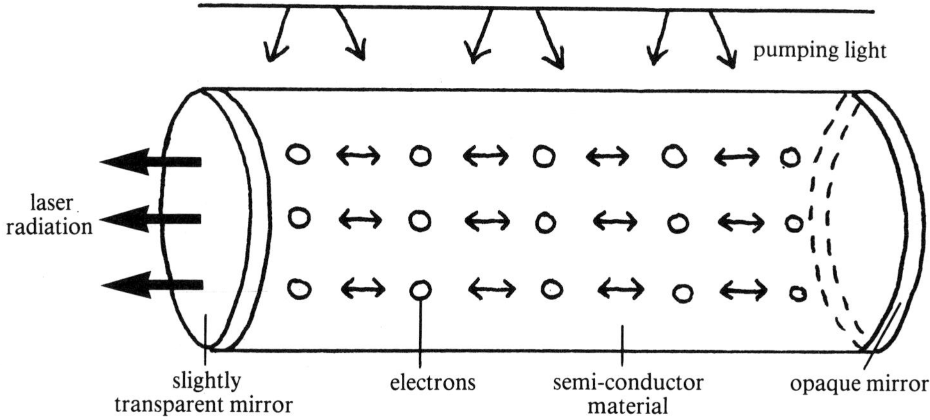

Figure 93. Diagram showing mechanism of laser emission.

of energy. This has the effect of pushing electrons out to an outer shell, and they thereby become unstable when situated in this shell. They tend to drop back to the lowest energy level at which their orbit is stable. This is illustrated by the Bohr model of the hydrogen atom (see Figure 94).

As the energized electrons drop down to their original stable level they emit a photon of energy. These photons travel backwards and forwards within the material used for laser action and are reflected from the mirrors at either end of the material. Soon all photons of the same wavelength resonate with one another, and a highly coherent beam of light is produced which escapes from the operating end of the laser through the mirror which is 95 per cent reflective. The wavelength of this beam of light determines as to whether the laser is in the near infra-red range; the infra red range, or the visible light range. Acupuncture lasers are produced in all these

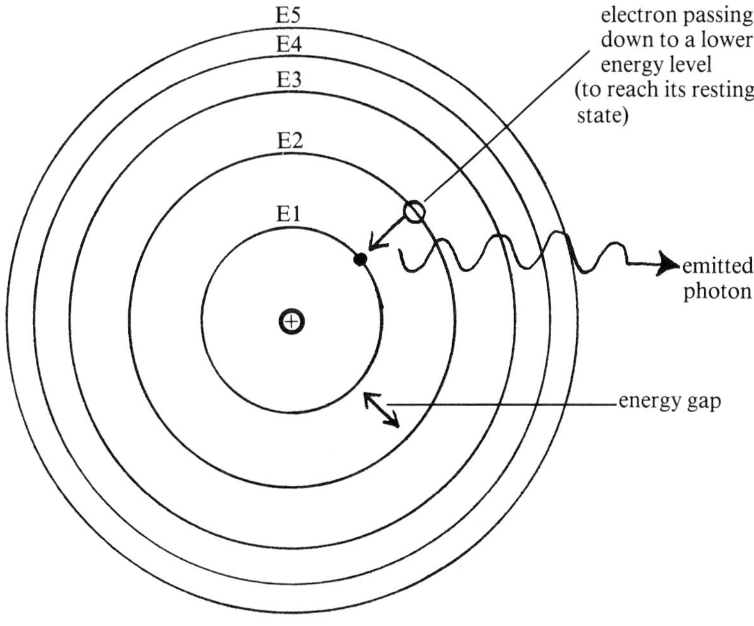

Figure 94. Bohr model of the hydrogen atom.

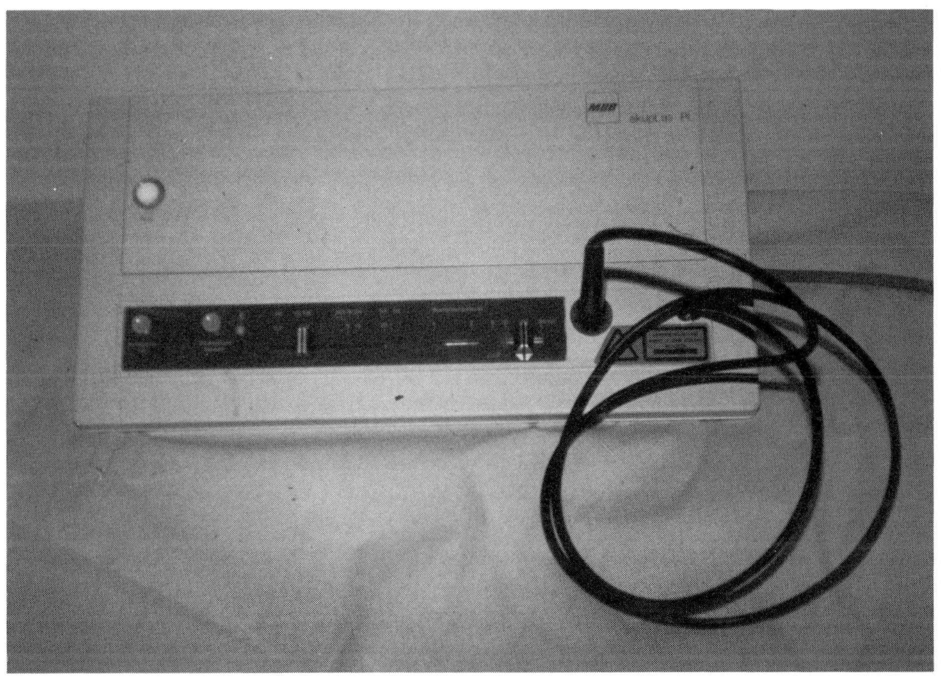

Figure 95. The *MBB Akuplas* laser.

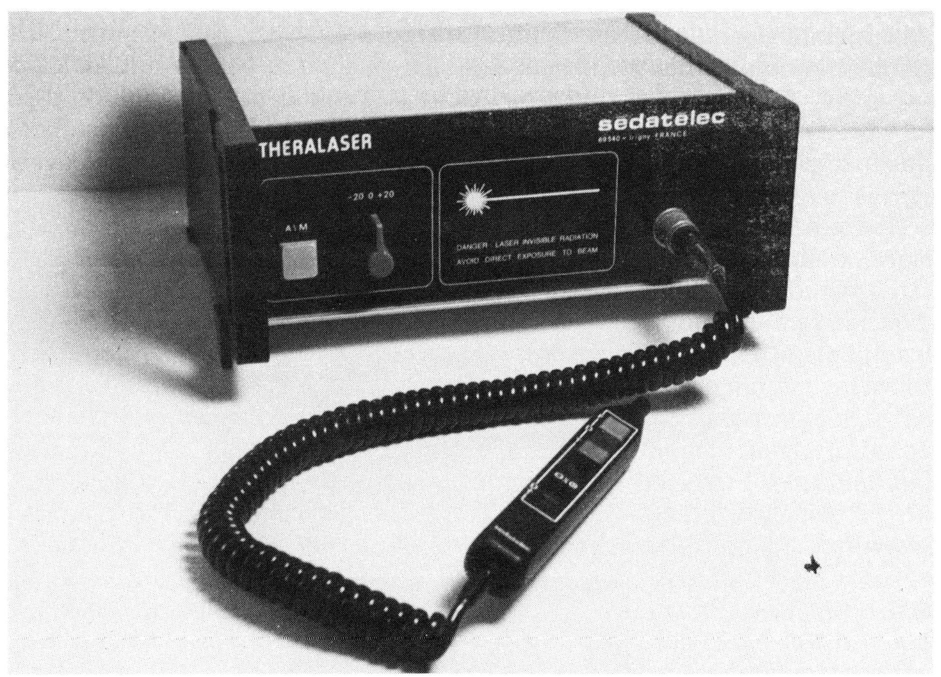

Figure 96. The *Theralaser DT*.

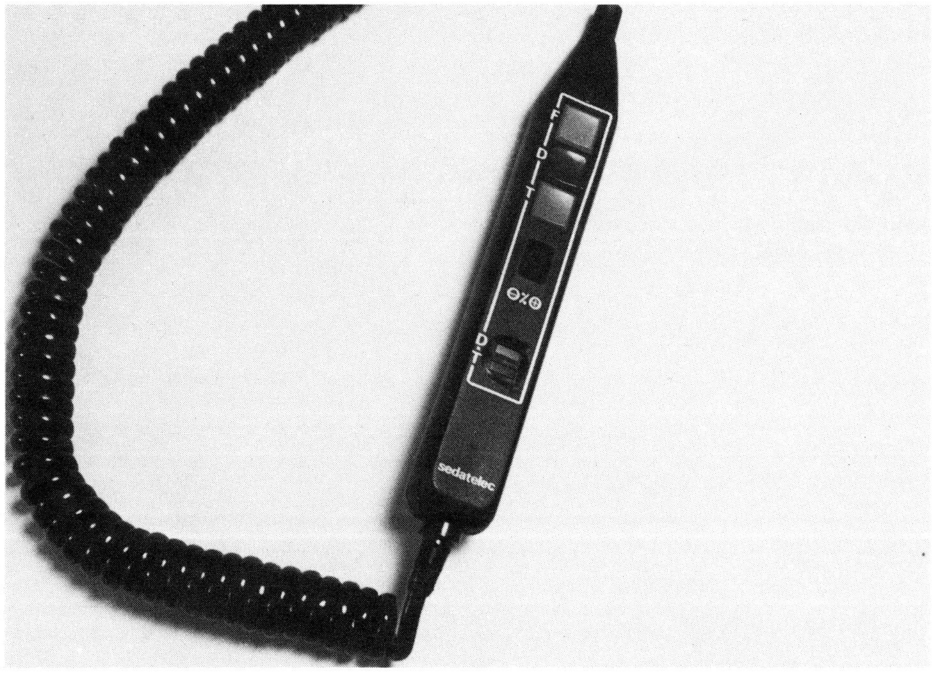

Figure 97. The treatment probe of the *Theralaser DT*.

ranges. The *Theralaser* produces radiation in the near infra red range which is invisible to the eye. The *MBB Akuplas* laser* produces radiation in the infra-red range, which is visible as a red beam, and the SVESA laser† produces a beam at a slightly higher frequency than infra-red, which is visible as a white beam.

All the lasers mentioned have a facility for modulating the frequency of the laser beam; this means that the laser beam can be oscillated, but this in no way changes the wavelength of the laser radiation. Only the *Theralaser* has a facility for modulating the laser radiation according to the seven frequencies corresponding to the seven ear zones, designated A, B, C, D, E, F, and G according to Nogier. The *MBB Akuplas* laser and the *Theralaser* are illustrated in Figures 95, 96 and 97.

Pathological points on the ear should be detected in the normal way. Whilst palpating the ACR the laser probe should be held over each point, firstly with frequency A modulating the laser beam with the diagnosis button depressed. This is illustrated in Figure 98.

The Use of the Laser in Auricular Therapy

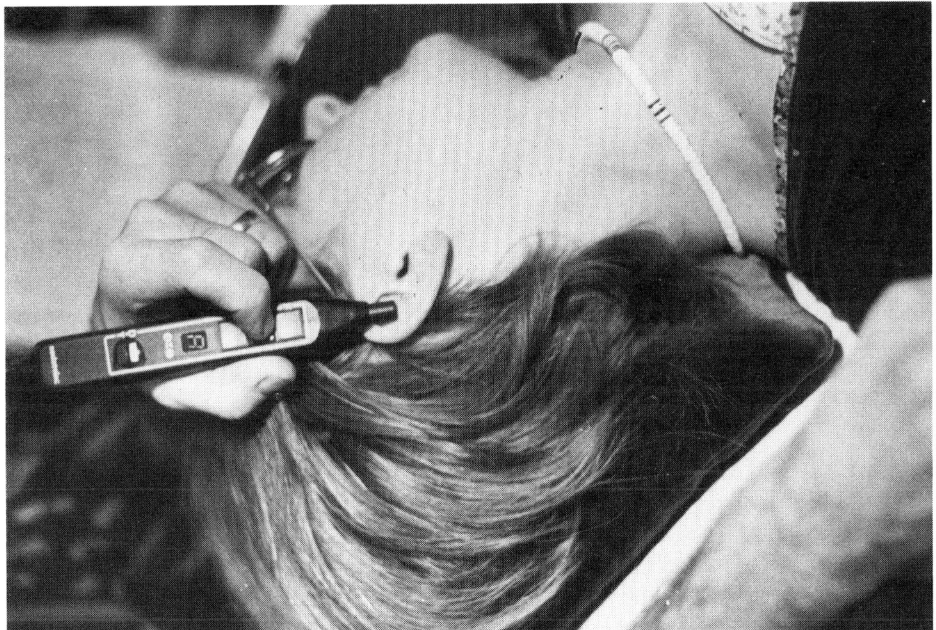

Figure 98.   Treatment of ear points using the *Theralaser DT*.

If any point is found to produce a positive ACR with the diagnosis button depressed with frequency A in operation, then the red therapy button should be depressed whilst holding the probe directly over the pathological point. On doing this the ACR quickly becomes negative, then it will slowly become positive again,

**MBB Akuplas* — manufactured by Messerschmitt — Bolkav — Blohm GmbH, POB 801149, D-8000, Munchen, West Germany.
†SVESA laser — Manufactured by SVESA GmbH, Otztalstr 7, 8 Munchen 70, West Germany.

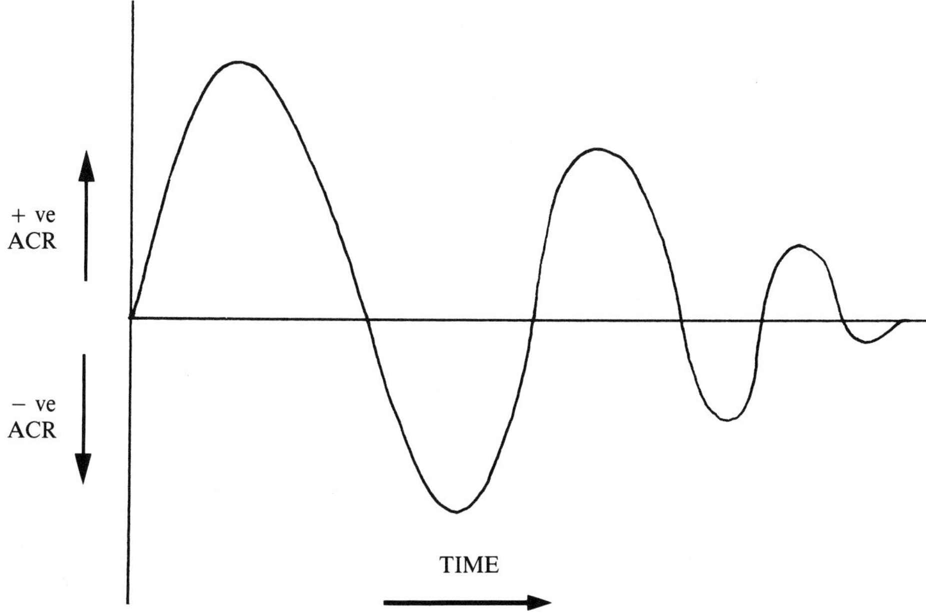

Figure 99.   Diagram showing damped oscillation reaction of ACR.

but not quite as positive as initially, and then it will become slightly less negative, until after approximately thirty seconds the pulse returns to normal. This is illustrated diagrammatically in Figure 99.

The body reacts to any incoming radiation, which includes laser radiation, with a damped oscillation. This explains why the ACR is initially positive on detection with the diagnosis button depressed. With the therapy button depressed the ACR becomes markedly negative then slightly positive, and then less slightly negative, and lastly a normal pulse returns. Only when the normal pulse returns can the point be considered as treated adequately. Following this the same procedure is repeated for frequency B and so on right through to frequency G and the points are treated in the same manner. Generally speaking if a point is present in a particular zone, then it will give a positive ACR to the appropriate frequency of that zone when this frequency is applied to it. In other words, if a point is detected in zone C, then a positive ACR will generally be obtained if C is dialled on the probe of the *Theralaser*. It is not uncommon to find a point resonating to two or three different frequencies; two of these frequencies will of course be different from the basic frequency of the zone in which the pathological point is situated. This occurrence is termed 'parasitage' by Nogier, and it is recommended that the zones corresponding to the parasite frequencies detected should also be searched with the diagnosis side of the laser probe, and in these zones, a positive ACR point will be found. Then these zones ought to be treated with their own particular frequency at the point so detected, the supposition being that these particular areas of the zones involved are 'parasiting' upon the original pathological point.

For example, if a point in zone C is found to give a positive ACR when the *Theralaser* with the diagnosis button is depressed and placed over that point to the frequencies C, E and F, this would indicate that frequencies E and F are parasitic frequencies on that point. Frequency C on that point would be expected as the point is situated in zone C. Therefore zone E should be searched with the probe of the *Theralaser* with frequency E operating with the diagnosis button depressed; a point in zone E will then yield a positive ACR. This should then be treated with the therapy button depressed, in exactly the same way as for any pathological point using E frequency. The same should be done for zone F. In the author's experience this is a useful therapeutic procedure and it is worth following through carefully. It will be clear from the above description that the diagnosis button on the *Theralaser* probe emits a very low powered beam, whereas the therapy button emits the highest power that the machine is capable of delivering.

It is recommended that lasers should never be directed at the cornea as there is a **Safety** possibility that cataract formation may occur. The safety of the *Akuplas* has been **Precautions with** tested on experimental animals by Bischko.[1] The animals (pigs) were irradiated for **Lasers** twenty-four hours with the probe of the *Akuplas* taped to the skin. This was done on a number of different sites on the pig's body. The sites were then examined, both by the naked eye and histologically, to see if any tissue damage had occurred. No tissue damage of any sort occurred. Bischko also used the same method on corneas of pigs to see if any adverse affects were produced; again, the *Akuplas* probe was directed at the cornea of the pig for twenty-four hours; again similar investigations were carried out, no adverse effects were noted. Therefore acupuncture lasers may be considered safe, yet the author considers it wise to observe the precaution of keeping the beam away from the patient's eyes.

A number of clinical trials have been conducted with the *Akuplas* apparatus. All **Clinical Trials** have concerned either classical acupuncture or wound healing. Hoffman[2] found **with Lasers** laser therapy on classical acupuncture points in children's complaints to be effective. Mester[3] found irradiation of wounds stimulated healing and Casper[4] found the best results were obtained with diseases related to the connective tissue, such as soft tissue rheumatism. It is clear from the work done on the application of lasers to classical acupuncture that the results are not as good as when traditional needling is used. This is presumably because most of the acupuncture points are situated beyond reach of the lasers used on classical acupuncture points. No properly conducted trial has yet been done on the use of laser therapy in auricular medicine. Clinically results are far superior to the use of laser on classical acupuncture points, perhaps because acupuncture points on the ear are situated close to the surface. This is emphasized by the finding that a very low power laser indeed, which is battery operated, (*GIR. 56*)* is sufficient in some cases to produce therapeutic effects on pathological points situated on the ear. The *GIR. 56* is used in exactly the same way as the *Theralaser*. Its advantage is that it is portable but a disadvantage is that it is a low powered device. It has both a diagnostic and a therapy button exactly as the *Theralaser*, and a rotating wheel for dialling in the appropriate Nogier frequency from A through to G (see Figure 100). The application of the *GIR. 56* in the auricular therapy on pathological ear points is illustrated in Figure 101.

**GIR. 56* manufactured by Sedatelec.

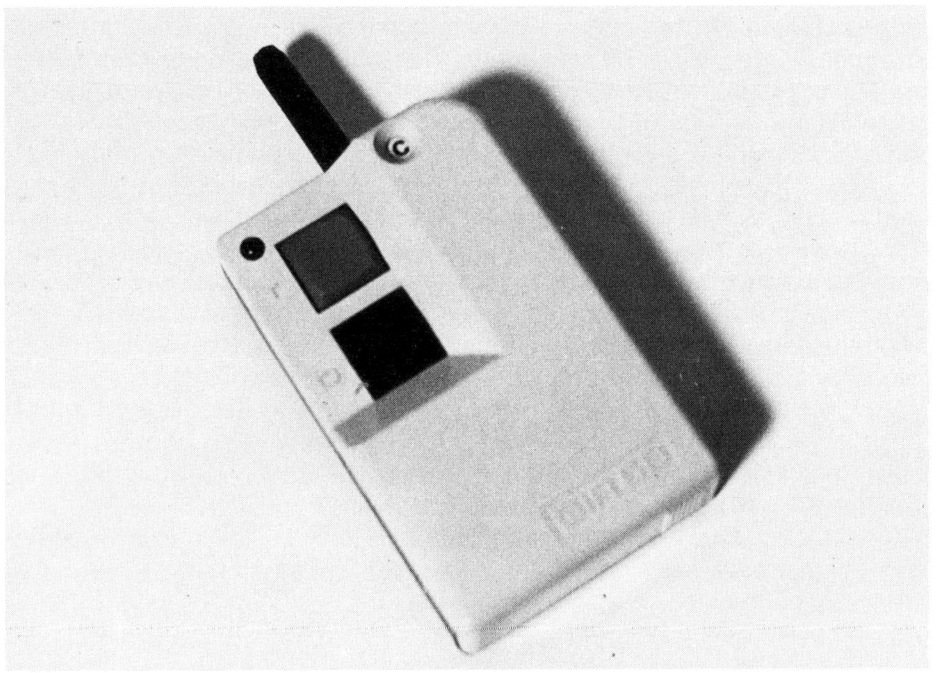

Figure 100.   The *GIR. 56.*

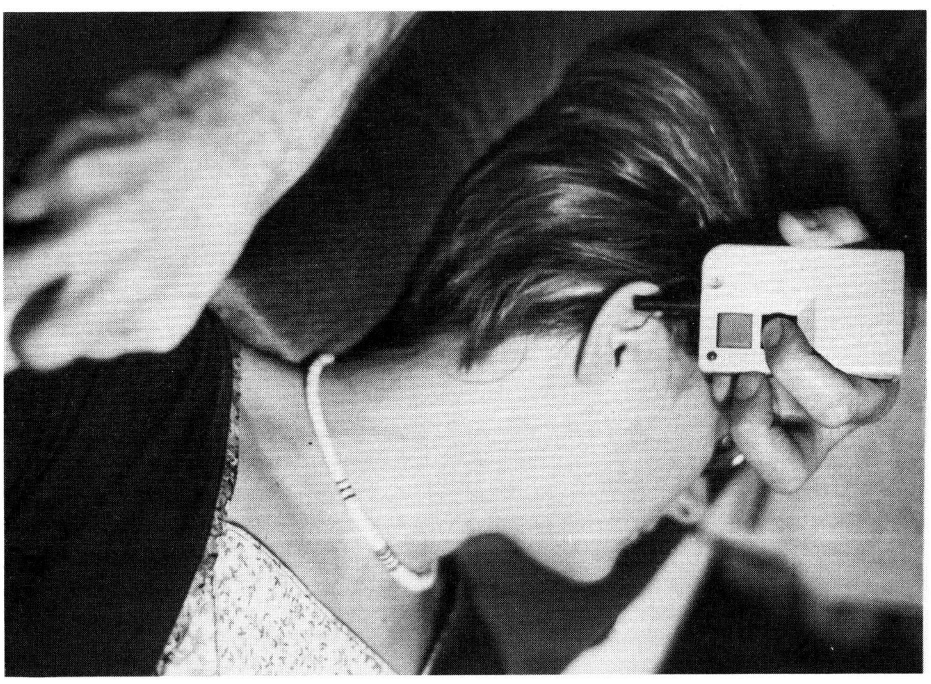

Figure 101.   Treatment of pathological points using the *GIR. 56.*

It is a pity that the *GIR. 56* is made only for right handed users; it is awkward to operate with the left hand due to the position of the wheel which dials in the different frequencies.

Laser therapy is effective and useful when applied in auricular therapy. It is less **Conclusion** effective than classical acpuncture for reasons stated above. Unfortunately there is no way of defining as to whether a pathological point is best treated with a laser or a magnetic field or with a needle. If and when such a question can be answered reliably, then laser therapy will be more effective, as its choice for use in any particular case can rest on a reasoned decision as to which form of energy the point is best treated by. At the moment, the application of laser energy tends to be trial and error.

The application of lasers to classical acupuncture and to auricular therapy will become more effective if lasers can be devised with a variable power output, and therefore, by inference, a greater or lesser depth of penetration; in other words a method for focusing on the acupuncture point. Also a device for varying the frequency of the radiation itself, from the near infra-red band through the visible light band and perhaps into the ultra-violet band may well render laser therapy more effective. As yet laser activity in the ultra-violet region has not been achieved, so this looks very much to the future, but remains a possibility.

The main technical difference between the three lasers discussed in this chapter are that they all emit laser radiation in different wavebands. Unfortunately it is not possible to ascertain as to which particular waveband of radiation is the best to use on acupuncture points. It is probably a stronger possibility that different acupuncture points require different wave lengths of applied radiation. In the author's view, as auricular therapy is the application of choice of laser therapy in its present stage of development, then the *Theralaser* is the preferable equipment, as the dialing of the Nogier frequency is facilitated by the frequency button on the probe, whereas on the SVESA laser and the *MBB Akuplas* laser an assistant is required in order to turn the frequency modulation of the laser beam through its range.

CHAPTER TWENTY

THERAPEUTIC APPLICATION OF MAGNETIC FIELDS

A number of different ways of applying magnetic fields in therapy are in general use amongst practitioners using acupuncture and auricular medicine. These are the application of pulsed magnetic fields (MF therapy), the application of a magnetic pole to pathological points (*Therapuncteur EMS.20*), and the application of either alternating fields or static fields across the cranium (*Theramagnetic*).

MF Therapy MF therapy is the application of pulsed magnetic fields to diseased areas. This is carried out using equipment called the *Biopulse** (see Figure 102). The magnetic field can be applied to the diseased area, either via a flat applicator, which is movable on a hinged arm (see Figure 103) or via a cylindrical applicator which is also supplied with a hinged arm system, and this is placed around the patient for treating conditions in the thorax or abdomen (see Figure 104). The only book available on MF therapy by Fichtner[1] gives a list of over eighty references, none of which specifically refer to any clinical trial of the application of pulsed magnetic fields to disease, other than referring to its use for bone healing. The usefulness of pulsed magnetic fields for any situation in which healing is required can be accepted as well proven. However, its application to disease in general cannot be regarded as proven, or even investigated at the present time. The book *MF Therapy* lists a series of conditions together with numbers of patients treated with percentage results obtained, these were compiled from practitioners using the *Biopulse* machine, and were obtained by the company manufacturing the *Biopulse* by a questionnaire sent out to practitioners who had purchased *Biopulse* machines. These figures therefore cannot be regarded as in any way reliable. The booklet then goes on to give advice on the frequency and strength in gauss of the applied field in different conditions. In the author's view there is no evidence available in the literature on frequency to indicate other than that low frequency fields of around ten cycles per second are probably more biologically effective than other frequencies. The MF therapy

**Biopulse* manufactured by Elec., Wiesbaden, West Germany.

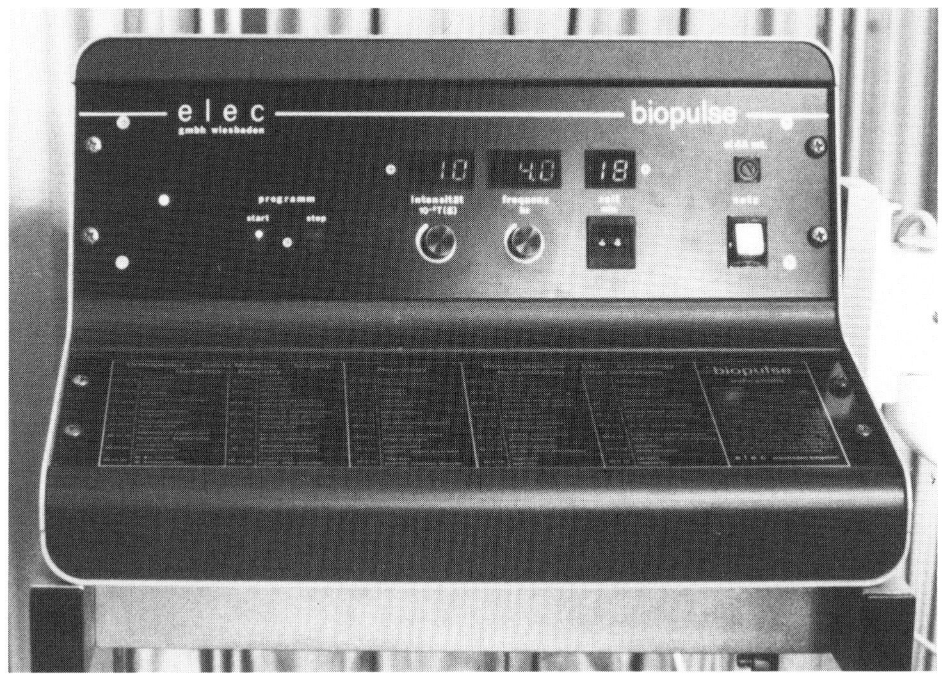

Figure 102.   The *Biopulse* control unit.

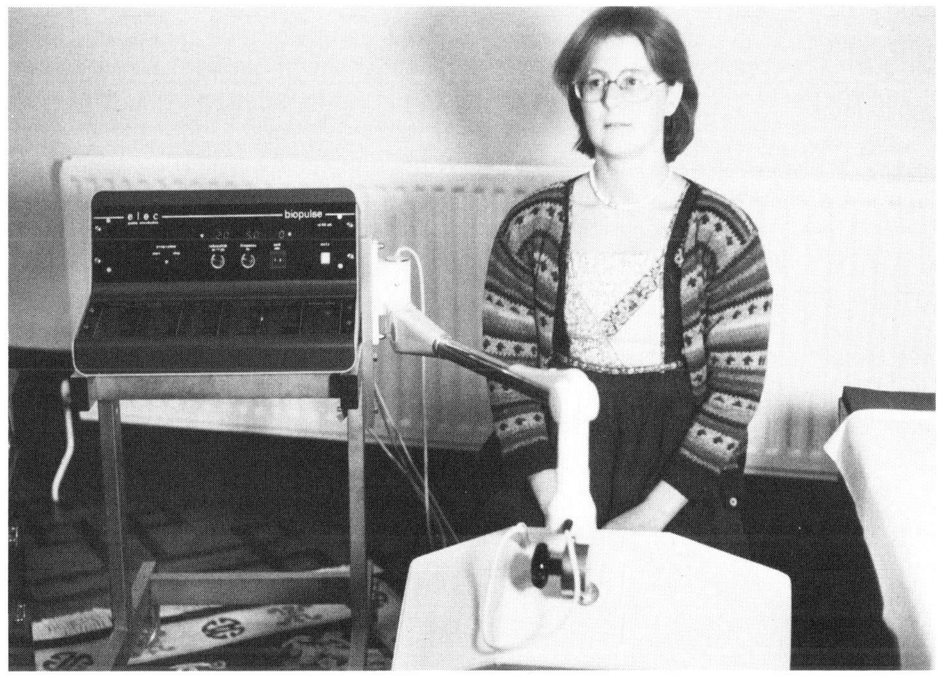

Figure 103.   Treatment with the flat applicator of the *Biopulse*.

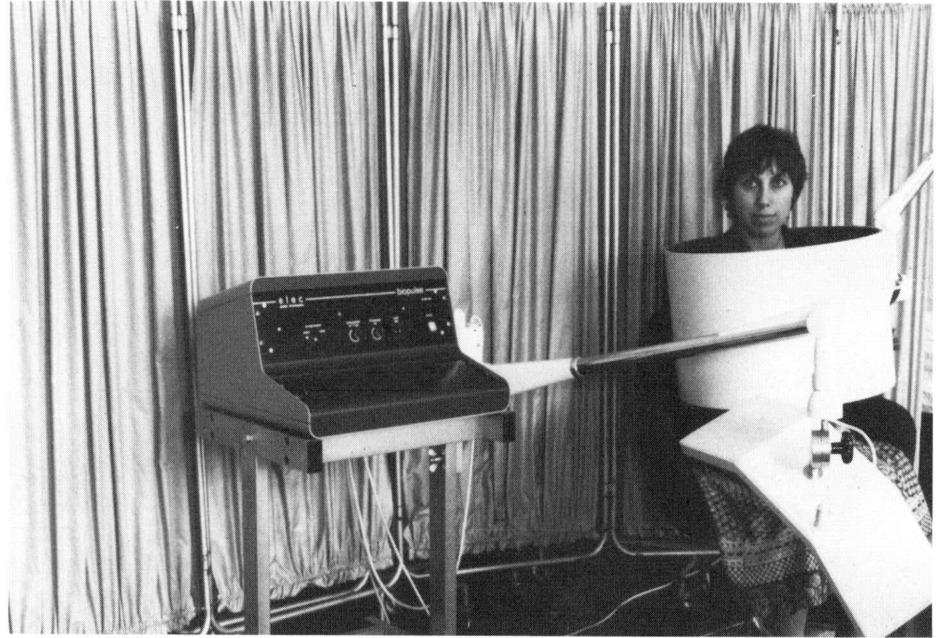

Figure 104.   Treatment with the cylindrical applicator of the *Biopulse.*

book gives a wide range of field strengths and frequencies which should be applied in different condition for which there is absolutely no evidence of any sort.

The author's practice is to place the applicator over the diseased part, and palpate the ACR. Switch the machine on and slowly turn up the strength of magnetic field (the *Biopulse* can deliver a magnetic field strength ranging from 1 to 100 gauss). When the ACR is maximal the strength of magnetic field is left at that level. Following this the same is done with the frequency dial (the *Biopulse* can deliver a pulsating magnetic field varying from 1 to 50 hertz). Initially sessions of twenty minutes are given and on each subsequent appointment a longer session is given. In general it appears better to start with low field strengths and to work up to higher field strengths towards the end of a course of treatment.

Using the ACR in this manner has shown that frequencies of field around about 10 hertz nearly always produce a positive ACR.

Results from treatment with pulsating magnetic fields, other than in fractures or situations where healing processes need to be stimulated such as an indolent ulcers, tend to be haphazard. The author has found the application of pulsed magnetic fields to be useful in cases of nerve damage, particularly peripheral neuropathy. Assessment in other areas of therapy such as chronic pain have been unclear and in the author's experience some patients have gained relief, while others have not; the problem being to determine as to whether application of pulsed magnetic fields is likely to produce a result or not in any particular patient. The answer to these questions will become clearer in the future as further research is undertaken.

The *Therapuncteur EMS.20* is a piece of equipment for applying either an electric field or a magnetic pole onto a pathological point. Facilities are included in the apparatus for oscillating the applied electric field, or magnetic pole at any of the seven Nogier frequencies A to G and also at a very slow frequency termed 'frequency U' which is called the 'universal frequency'. This frequency is supposed to be useful for all pathological points, or in situations where a choice of frequency is unclear. In these situations, frequency U should be applied. The equipment is illustrated in Figure 105.

The Therapuncteur EMS.20*

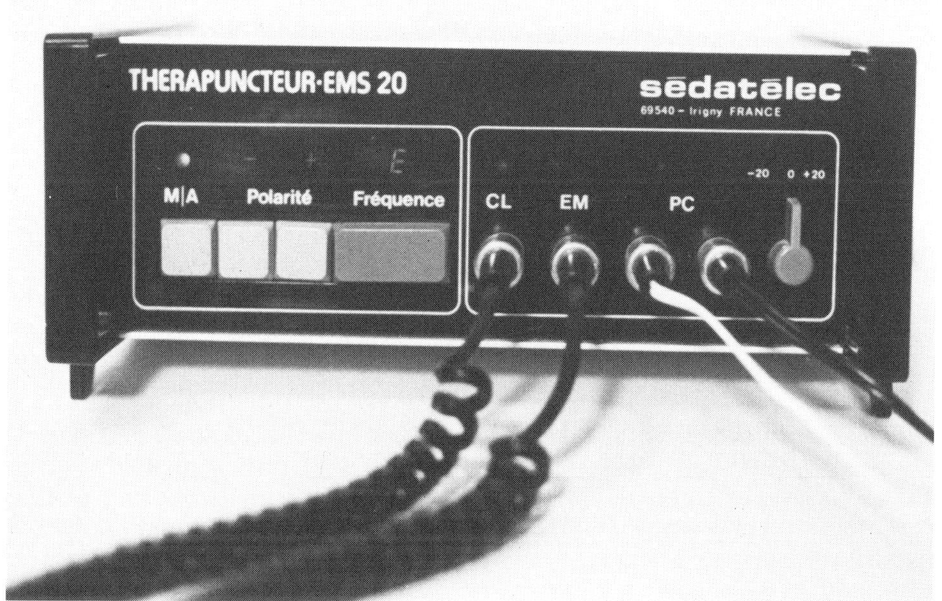

Figure 105. The *Therapuncteur EMS.20.*

A flashing light-emitting diode is provided as a diagnostic aid on the *EMS.20*, and this flashes on and off in time with the frequency that the equipment is delivering at that particular moment. This is used over pathological points in order to determine the frequency of applied stimulation, either magnetic or electric, and corresponds to the diagnostic side of the *Theralaser* (see Figure 111).

The polarity buttons (+ and −) can either be pressed in separately or together. If the polarity buttons are pressed in separately, then either a positive or negative electric field, depending on which button is pressed, is projected at the end of the electric probe (see Figure 106), or a north pole (negative − ve button on *EMS.20*), or a south pole (positive + ve button on the *EMS.20*) is projected onto the end of the magnetic probe (see Figure 106). As indicated earlier, both the magnetic and electric fields can be oscillated at frequencies A to G and also the universal frequency U. If both positive and negative buttons are depressed simultaneously, then an alternating magnetic or electric field is produced at the tip of the appropriate probe.

**Therapuncteur EMS.20* manufactured by Sedatelec.

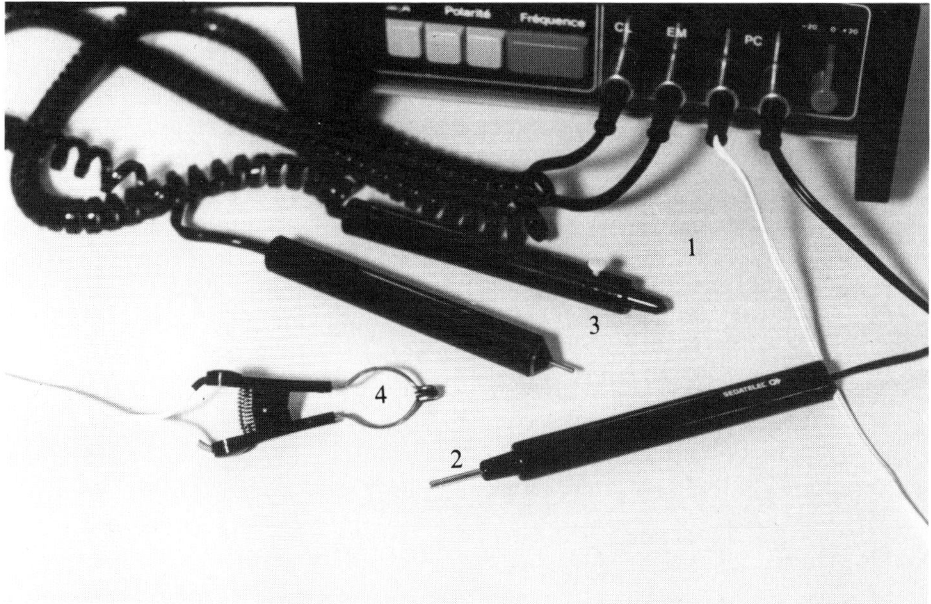

Figure 106.   Flashing diode (1) electric (2) magnetic (3) and spring clip applicator (4) probes for the *Therapuncteur EMS.20.*

A springloaded clip is also supplied with the *EMS.20* with an electric field of positive polarity projected onto one side, and an electric field of opposite polarity projected onto the other side of the clip. This can be applied to the ear over pathological points as an alternative means of applying an electric field to a pathological point.

The Use of the Therapuncteur EMS.20

In order to apply an electric field to a pathological point, point detection is carried out in the normal way, and if the point gives a positive reaction to the positive side of the positive/negative hammer (or to the black side of the black/white hammer, or to the gold side of the gold/silver hammer, black and positive = gold needle), then a positive field should be applied at the spring-loaded electric probe. This is applied directly onto the pathological point, and held using light pressure until the ACR becomes normal (see Figure 107). If the point requires a negative electric field, then the opposite field is applied.

An alternative method of applying an electric field to a point can be achieved by applying the clip over the pathological point. The clip is attached to the ear with the positive side placed directly over the point, if a positive electric field is needed for therapy (i.e. detection with positive side of positive/negative hammer etc.). This therefore means that the negative side of the clip is present on the opposite side of the ear. The opposite procedure is carried out if the point requires a negative electric field. This is illustrated in Figure 108. The clip is left on the point until the ACR returns to a normal pulse.

The electric side of the *EMS.20* and the clip applicator of this electric field as discussed above, is a useful method of correcting disordered electric laterality. This

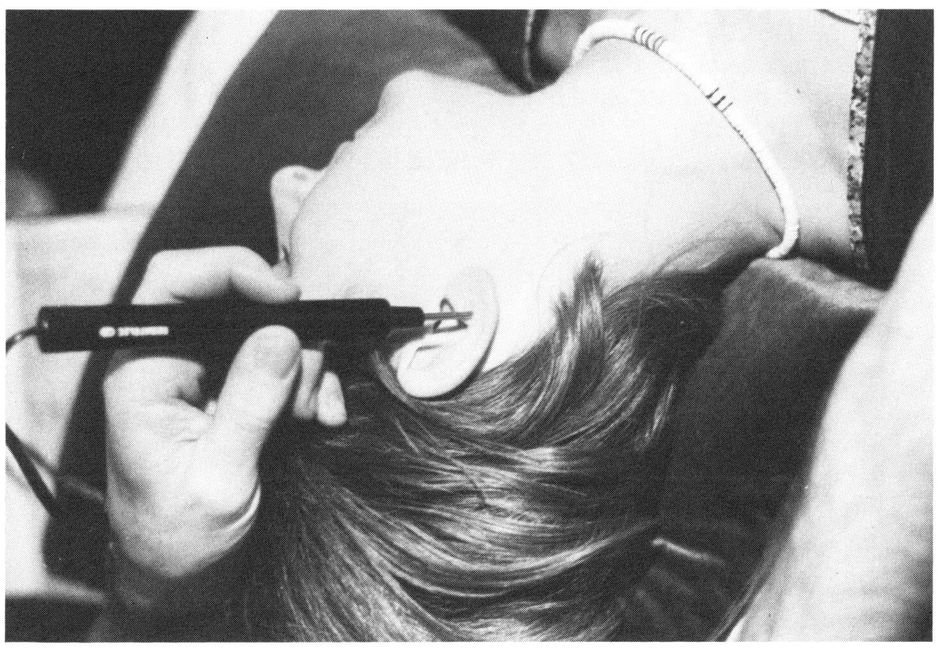

Figure 107. Treatment of a pathological point using the electric probe.

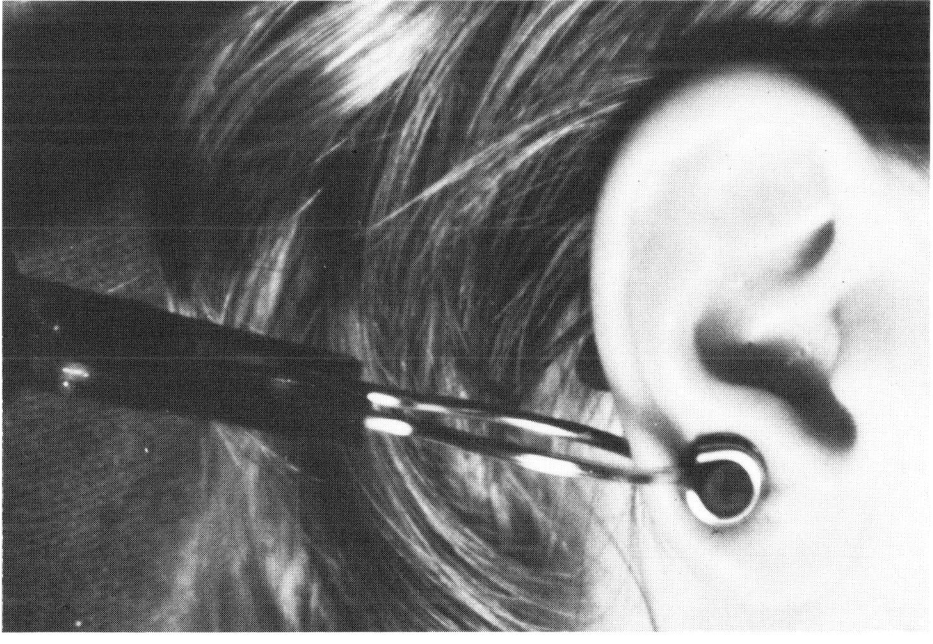

Figure 108. The application of an electric field to a pathological point via the spring clip applicator.

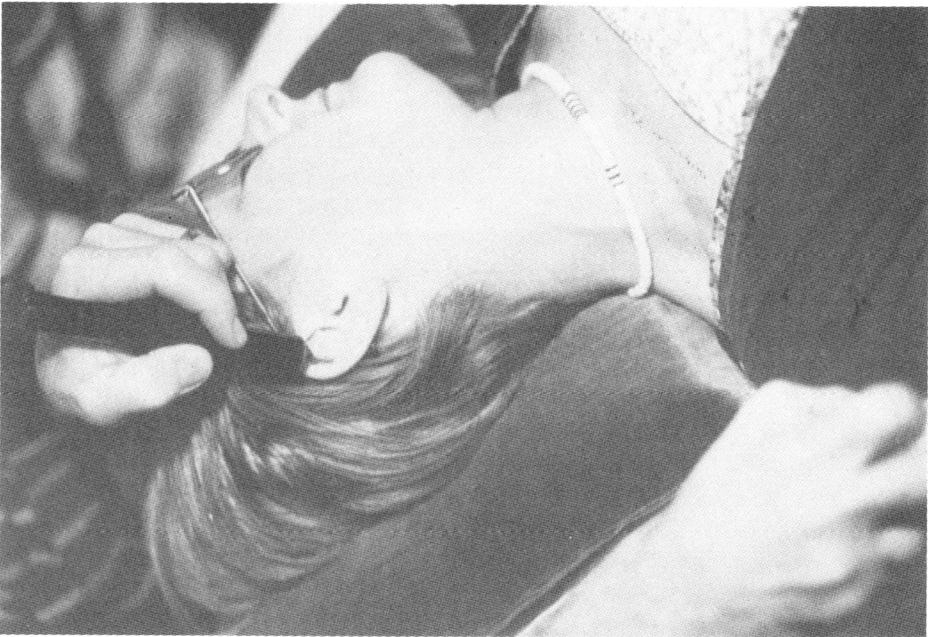

Figure 112. Application of the magnetic pole of the *EMS.20* to a pathological ear point.

pole. However, on the *Therapuncteur* the south pole is obtained by pressing the positive button, and the north pole is obtained by pressing the negative button. This is an apparent contradiction, and the reason for it is that black and positive detection means that a north pole or a gold needle is required. In order to produce this effect the opposite pole needs to be projected onto the point because, as with the projection of any magnetic field, a dipole effect occurs. Therefore, in order to produce a north pole on a point, a south pole needs to be projected from the equipment. To make things simpler from the therapeutic point of view detection with the positive side of the positive/negative hammer means that the positive button of the *EMS.20* should be depressed, and this in turn will project a south pole which will then cause a north pole to form on the pathological point, in exactly the same way as if a bar magnet was placed near to a piece of unmagnetized metal then the metal would become magnetized under the influence of the bar magnet with the opposite pole to the nearest pole of the bar magnet forming in the originally non-magnetized piece of metal. Exactly the same happens over a pathological point. The opposite pertains when a south pole is required on a pathological point.

The appropriate frequency of the magnetic field is determined according to the maximal positive ACR to the light-emitting diode, exactly as with the use of the diagnostic side of the *Theralaser*.

If the detection of a pathological point is unclear, in other words when it is not clear whether the point is giving a positive ACR to the positive or negative side of the positive/negative hammer, an alternating field ought to be applied at the tip of the treatment probe by depressing both the positive and negative buttons simultaneously. This is exactly the same situation as needling a pathological point with stainless steel, as opposed to gold and silver, when a similar diagnostic situation arises. As with all other treatment of pathological points therapy is continued until the ACR returns to a normal pulse.

On both the *Theralaser* and the *Therapuncteur EMS.20* there is a facility for slight increase or decrease of each of the Nogier frequencies. This is accomplished by a red switch which can be either switched to the right; this increases the frequency being beamed by the instrument by 20 per cent, or to the left, which decreases the frequency by 20 per cent. This can be regarded as a fine tuning of the frequency applied to a point. Nogier teaches that if the point has been detected by the white side of the black/white hammer, and thereby by inference, the silver side of the gold/silver hammer or the negative side of the positive/negative hammer, then the frequency ought to be increased by 20 per cent; in other words the switch ought to be pushed to the right. Conversely, if the point is detected with the black side of the black/white hammer, or the positive side of the positive/negative hammer etc., then the switch should be pushed to the left, and the frequency decreased by 20 per cent. More recent pieces of equipment, particularly the newer versions of the *GIR* have a facility for altering the basic frequency by plus or minus 30.

In the author's view this slight change of frequency, when applied to a point, is theoretically important in that it should be possible to obtain a bigger resonance effect, and therefore a bigger initial ACR when treating the pathological point, but in terms of results it is difficult to ascertain as to whether changing the frequency by plus or minus 20 per cent has any significant effect on therapy, and this must at the moment remain an open question until tested in a properly controlled manner.

Theramagnetic

The *Theramagnetic* is an apparatus which applies a magnetic field across the cranium, with an ability to project a strong, or a weak field of north or south on either ear, or an alternating field oscillating north/south, south/north etc., across the cranium. A new development of the *Theramagnetic* has been the inclusion of crossed polaroids which can be rotated through 360° over both poles of the electromagnet. This piece of equipment is termed the *Theramagnetic-P** and represents a big step forward in terms of therapeutic effect. The phenomenon of so-called 'polarized magnetism' or 'reticular energy' will be discussed in detail in the following chapter. The discussion here will be confined to instructions for use of the *Theramagnetic* in a clinical situation. It is recommended that the *Theramagnetic-P* is obtained as this can be dismantled in order to produce a simple *Theramagnetic* without the polaroid ear pieces on, and therefore this equipment represents a more versatile machine (see Figures 113 and 114).

It will be noted that a frame with the electrodes on moveable rails is illustrated. Another method of applying the electrodes is by means of earphones which are available either with or without polaroids. In the author's view the earphones are less versatile than the frame as illustrated in Figure 113 and the only advantage that the earphones with magnetic poles have is greater ease of application, and the patient is able to walk around with the equipment during therapy. But, as therapy only carries on for at the most ten minutes, the earphones are not really necessary.

**Theramagnetic-P* manufactured by Sedatelec.

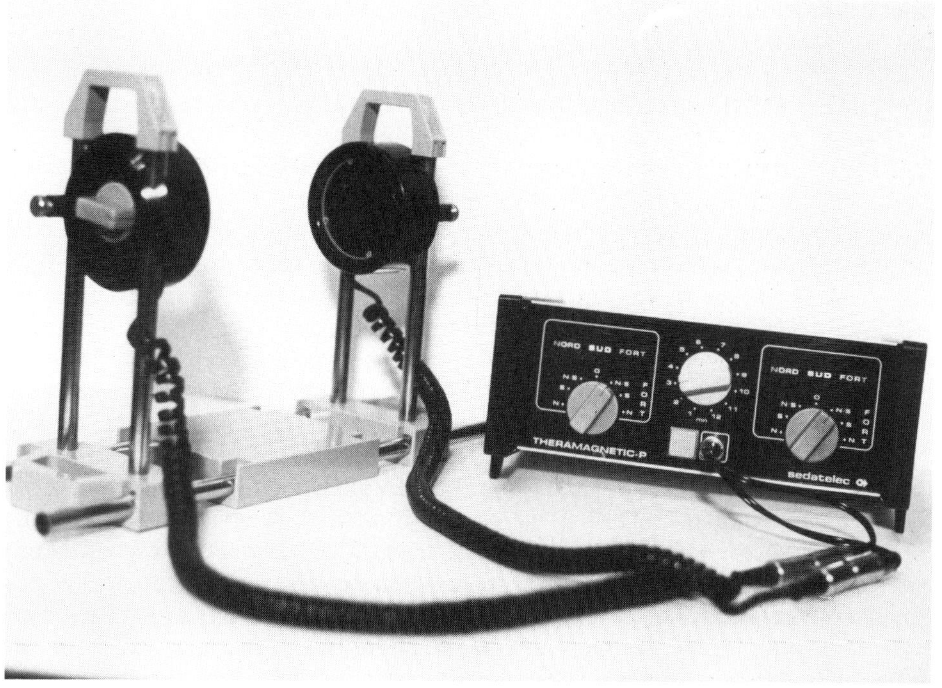

Figure 113. The *Theramagnetic-P* with the electrodes on a sliding frame.

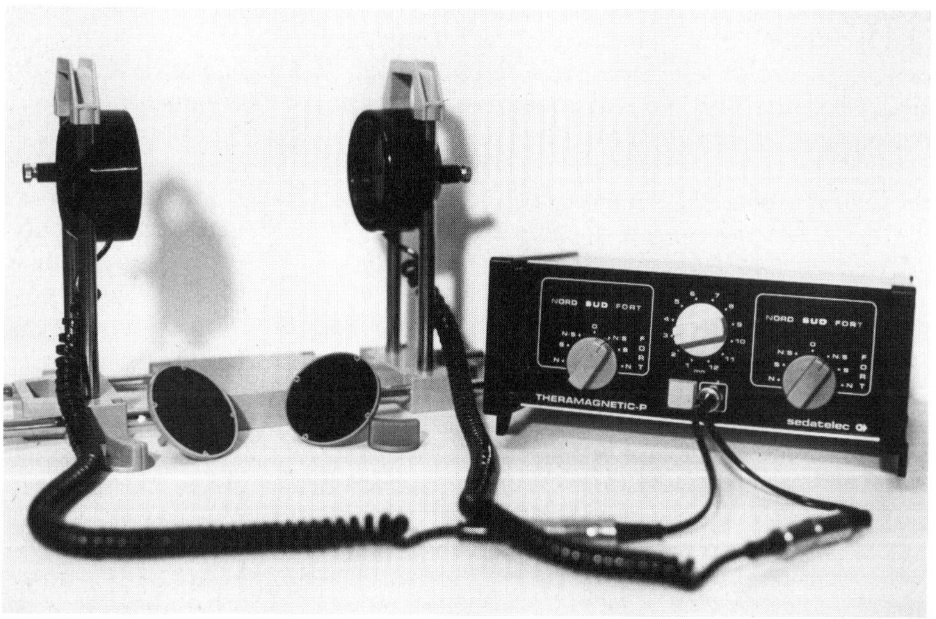

Figure 114. The *Theramagnetic-P* with the polaroid ear pieces removed.

Uses of the *Theramagnetic*

The *Theramagnetic* can be used to correct inversion. Inversion is a condition in which the sympathetic and parasympathetic areas of the body react the opposite way to their normal reaction; in other words the skin over the cheek responds as if it were sympathetic, and the skin over the arm responds as if it were parasympathetic. The detection of this situation is carried out by means of Noradrenaline and Acetylcholine ampoules, and this has been outlined in Chapter 10. In order to correct this situation an alternating strong magnetic field should be applied across both ears for approximately two minutes. This is illustrated in Figure 115. An alternating magnetic field applied across the cranium will obliterate all information gained from the ACR concerning allergy. Therefore, under no circumstances should a magnetic field of any sort, particularly an alternating magnetic field, be applied before allergy testing.

The teaching of the auriculotherapists regarding other applications of the *Theramagnetic* in different clinical situations tends to be contradictory and confusing, in that generally speaking a different answer is obtained from whichever authority is consulted. Some general rules emerge, and these therefore represent a consensus of opinion concerning applications of the *Theramagnetic* which can be carried out in practice with a reasonable hope of some therapeutic benefit arising.

The application of the *Theramagnetic* in the situation of inversion as detailed above, is one of these general rules, and this must be carried out prior to any therapy. If inversion has not been corrected after this procedure has been carried out, as determined by reaction to Noradrenaline and Acetylcholine ampoules, then therapy must be continued for a further period of time, until correction has been achieved.

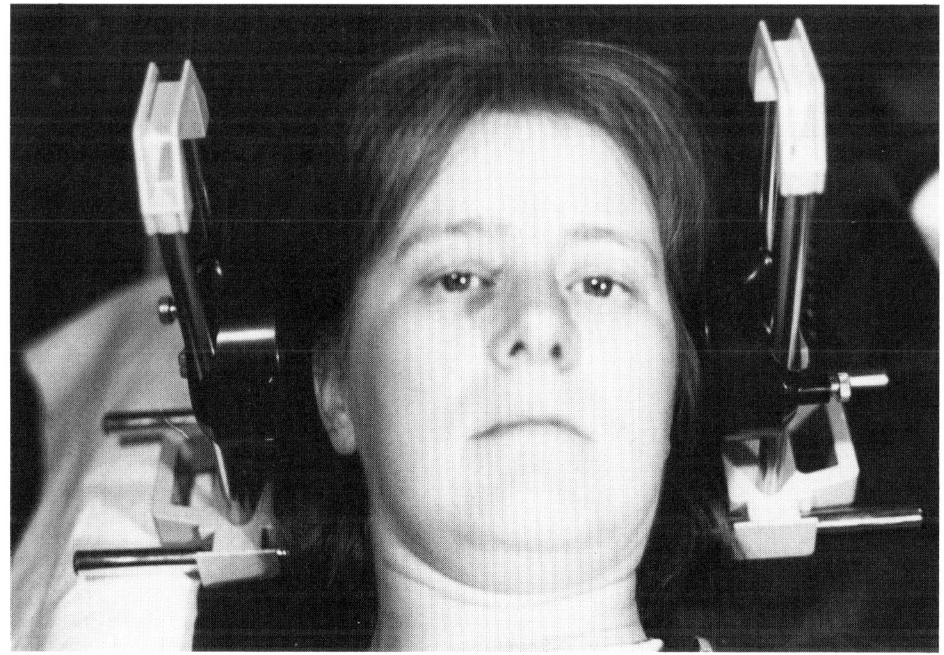

Figure 115.   The application of the *Theramagnetic* to a patient.

The *Theramagnetic-P* may be applied over gold and silver needles, in place on the ear by using an alternating polarized magnetic field for approximately three minutes whilst the needles are in place. This is a method of stimulating the needles whilst in place, even though the patient will derive no sensation from it. This leads to greater effectiveness of gold and silver needle therapy when applied to pathological points. In the author's experience no similar benefit is obtained using polarized magnetic fields over ears which have been previously treated using the laser on pathological points.

Two situations in which there is general agreement that the *Theramagnetic* ought to be used, concern so called 'disordered magnetic laterality' and 'disordered reticular laterality'. The concept of magnetic and reticular laterality will be discussed in detail in the following chapter. Their correction is outlined here, and concerns exclusively the use of the *Theramagnetic*. In disordered magnetic laterality the plain *Theramagnetic* should be used; in this case, the polaroid attachments to the earpieces should be removed, as shown in Figure 114. In a right-handed individual the south pole should be projected onto the right ear, and the north pole onto the left ear. A strong field should be applied. This ought to be carried out for a period of three minutes, after which detection to ascertain as to whether magnetic laterality has been corrected should be checked. If it is still abnormal, then further treatment with the *Theramagnetic* should be given. In the case of disordered reticular laterality a polarized strong magnetic field, with the north pole over the right ear of a right-handed patient, and the south pole over the left ear should be applied for a period of three minutes, and then detection should be carried out in exactly the same way. If further therapy is needed this can be instituted as appropriate.

A number of other confusing indications for the use of the *Theramagnetic* are taught. All of the above procedures, except the application of an alternating polarized magnetic field over needles in place in the ears should be applied prior to therapy, as it is likely that therapy will be more effective if carried out after the above procedures, if they are indicated. In any other situation the author's practice is to use the ACR in order to determine what sort of field is required. This is done by using the ACR, and switching one pole off; that is to zero position on the controls of the *Theramagnetic-P*, then the pole under investigation is turned on to weak north, and weak south, alternating weak north/south, then on to strong north and strong south and alternating strong north/south until the strongest positive ACR is obtained in one of these six positions. If no ACR occurs at any of these positions then the polaroid part of the earpiece should be removed, and the procedure carried out with plain poles in place over the patient's ears.

Once the setting of one side has been determined exactly the same procedure is carried out for the opposite side. Having therefore determined appropriate therapy, using the ACR as a biological measure, this can be applied in the usual way. The author's practice is to go through this procedure if no indications for specific use of the *Theramagnetic* as outlined above are required; in other words, in cases where reticular and magnetic laterality is normal and where there is no inversion.

Post-therapy, with needles in place, the author's practice is to always go through the procedure as outlined here, using the ACR to determine the appropriate settings of the *Theramagnetic*, then this is applied for three minutes as a general rule. The author's clinical findings are that this produces better results, and it is a sensible way of choosing what sort of field needs to be applied. It is not unusual to find that a south field needs to be projected on both ears, or a north field on both ears. Any combination is possible, and if indicated by the ACR it should be applied.

In order to treat a point with a polarized magnet, either a *Polatron North* or *Polatron South* should be used,* or a polarized magnet may easily be made by applying two pieces of polaroid, one at right angles to the other over each pole of a strong bar magnet. As strong a magnet as possible should be used. The pathological point will have been diagnosed in the usual way.

Treatment of Pathological Points Using Polarized Magnets

If on detection the point gave a position ACR either to the black side of the black/white hammer, or the positive side of the positive/negative hammer, then the point should be treated with a polarized north pole. This is done by using the ACR and passing the polarized north pole of the bar magnet over the pathological point until a maximum ACR is obtained. The ACR will soon become markedly negative, and then slightly positive again; in other words, a damped oscillation will occur in much the same way as the body responds to treatment when a laser is used.

If the point has been detected with the white side of the black/white hammer or the negative side of the positive/negative hammer then a polarized south pole should be used in exactly the same manner. If a *Polatron North* or *South* is used, then this is passed over the point in exactly the same way, and the handle on the *Polatron* should be depressed prior to treatment. This brings the crossed polaroids into line with either the north or south pole, depending on whether the *Polatron South* or *North* is being used. Nogier claims that all pathology which is extending deep in to the body's energy 'envelopes' needs to be treated with polarized magnetism. Unfortunately it is not possible to determine whether any particular pathological point will do better treated with polarized magnets or lasers or needles etc.

The author's practice has been to treat all the points on the ear either using needles or laser or the *Therapuncteur EMS.20* and then to leave the patient for five or ten minutes and then go over the ear again using the original detection method. If any point has reappeared, then this point is presumed to be the point representing the 'deepest pathology' and should be treated with a polarized magnet, or a small permanent magnet with either one or two sheets of polaroid glued on (Figure 116) can be placed over the point with the polaroid next to the skin. For this purpose, the magnet in the end of the semi-permanent needle dispenser is used. Making such a magnet is illustrated in Figure 116. It is applied to the pathological point which first returns on re-examining the ear by using appropriate sticking plaster as illustrated in Figure 117.

In the author's experience the application of this small polarized magnet produces marked clinical effects in certain patients. Unfortunately, when the magnet is removed symptoms often return. The author has studied a series of ten such patients, all with multiple food allergies. All of these patients' allergies could be controlled by placing a permanent polarized magnet on a point situated behind the earlobe. This point is designated 'omega main' by the auricular therapists. This name has no special meaning, but merely designates this particular point. The reason for this point being important in allergies is unclear. In all of the ten patients studied, when

Polatron North and *Polatron South* manufactured by Sedatelec.

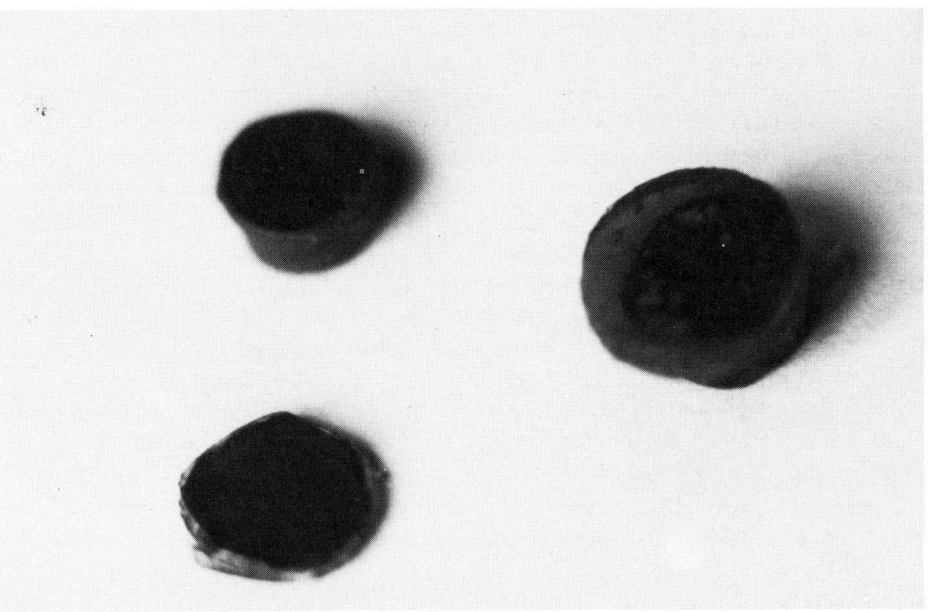

Figure 116. Preparation of a polarized permanent magnet showing the small disc magnet taken from the end of a semi-permanent needle holder and a circle of polaroid (on the left). These are glued together to make a polarized magnet as shown above (on the right).

the polarized magnet was removed, the symptoms gradually returned over a period varying between two to ten days. On replacing the magnet with a small brass disc with no polaroid filter on, no improvement occurred in any of the patients, but when this was substituted for a polarized magnet improvement occurred. Improvement, but to a much lesser extent, occurred when a permanent magnet without any polaroid filter attached was applied to the ear at the same point. The application of a polarized magnet to the point used in the treatment of patients with multiple allergies is illustrated in Figure 117. Usually the magnet will remain in place for between two to three weeks, and has been used by the author as an alternative to standard food dilution desensitization for food and chemical sensitivities. This method has been successful in some patients with other conditions such as chronic pain, and in a number of cases the polarized magnet has produced better results than either needles, lasers or the *Therapuncteur EMS.20*. The reasons for this are unclear, but exactly the same method was adopted in that the pathological points were treated, and then the ear was re-examined some five to ten minutes later. Then the points which reappeared (which were assumed to represent the deepest pathology in that particular patient), indicated with a permanent polarized magnet. In the author's experience the increase in effect from placing more than one sheet of polaroid over this small magnet did not appear to be clinically significant.

Another method of treating the point representing the deepest pathology as detected according to the method outlined above is to place a semi-permanent needle in this point. Insertion of semi-permanent needles has been described in Chapter 9. The semi-permanent needle applies strong stimulation to such a point, and in situations where a permanent polarized magnet is difficult to affix, such as over the edge of the helix, a semi-permanent needle can be usefully inserted.

The magnet supplied at the end of the semi-permanent needle holder ought to be rotated in a forwards direction over the needle. This ought to be done at least three times a day for approximately thirty seconds each time. The magnet need not touch the needle, but the direction of rotation of the magnet should be in a clockwise direction over the right ear, and an anti-clockwise direction over the left ear; in other words, always in a forwards direction. This will involve 're-cocking' the hand after each forward rotation of the magnet, and this is done by the patient drawing the stimulating hand away, re-cocking the magnet, and then approaching the semi-permanent needle again, and rotating once more in a forwards direction.

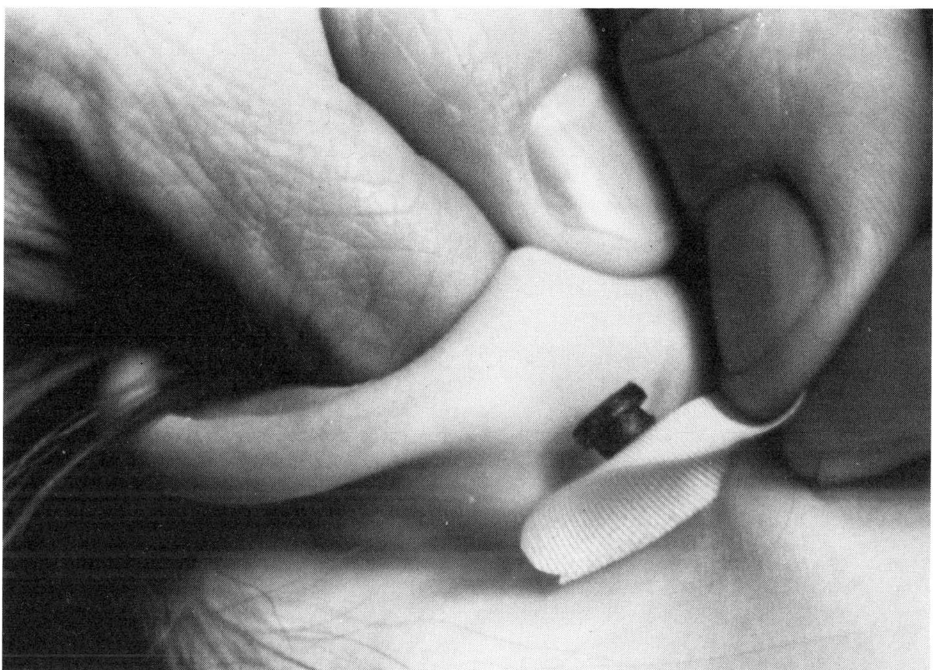

Figure 117.   The application of a polarized permanent magnet to a point behind the ear lobe in a patient with multiple allergies.

CHAPTER TWENTY-ONE

NEW CONCEPTS IN AURICULAR MEDICINE

A number of important new concepts are described by Nogier. As mentioned in the introduction to the section on auricular therapy and auricular medicine, many of these concepts tend to be complicated, confusing and often contradictory. However, a number are important and have a bearing on the success or otherwise of treatments via the ear.

All experienced practitioners in auricular medicine should be aware of these new concepts and be able to apply them in a practical situation.

Reticular Energy (Polarized Magnetism)

Nogier claims to have discovered a new form of energy which he terms 'reticular energy' or 'polarized magnetism'. This energy is produced by applying a sheet of linear polaroid over a magnetic pole. The strength of this energy is augmented by placing a second, or even a third piece of polaroid at right angles to the previous polaroid overlying the magnetic pole. Many claims are made for the therapeutic efficiency of so-called 'polarized magnetism'. An instrument for delivering this energy onto a pathological point is manufactured by Sedatelec and called the *Polatron*. Two *Polatrons* are available, one with twelve sheets of polaroid, each at an angle of 30° to the next sheet placed over a north pole of a strong bar magnet, and a similar piece of equipment with twelve crossed polaroids applied over a south pole. The application of the polaroid filters to the *Theramagnetic*, the so-called *Theramagnetic-P* has been mentioned in the previous chapter.

Claims have been made that the effect of polaroid when applied to a magnetic pole is to concentrate the magnetic flux, in that instead of the flux curving and returning to the opposite pole of the magnet, the magnetic flux is claimed to pass like a beam from the pole of the magnet over which polaroids have been placed. This effect is claimed to increase with the greater number of polaroid sheets applied to the magnetic pole, providing these sheets are placed at an angle to each other. It is presumed that if more than twelve crossed sheets are placed then no further increase of this so-called reticular energy is achieved.

In clinical practice there appears to be little doubt that applying polaroids to a magnetic pole increases the therapeutic efficiency of magnetism. So far it has only been possible to demonstrate this by finding patients who in the first place respond to reticular energy when applied over a pathological point, and subsequently treating these points using a brass bar instead of a magnet, and noting any difference in clinical result.

Experience shows that only a certain proportion of patients respond to this form of therapy. The reasons for this are unclear. An interesting study has been carried out by Rouxeville[1] who has found that if patients are studied with joint pathology, such as an osteoarthritic knee and if the cranium is placed in an alternating magnetic field, firstly, without polaroid filters, and then with polaroid filters applied over the magnetic poles, such as in the *Theramagnetic-P*, then when the plain magnetic field is applied the temperature of the skin over the pathological joint showed an average rise of 0.3°C during the first three minutes of application of the field. However, if a polarized magnetic field is applied, then the average temperature rise over the joint in a series of fifty patients was found to be 1.2°C. The author has confirmed this phenomena, together with Rouxeville. These findings, although confirmed, were not carried out under laboratory conditions. This is of some importance as measurement of changes in skin temperature requires a controlled environment as the results are prone to artefact.

Melville and Lewith[2] have investigated the effects of polaroid filters on magnetic fields at the request of the author, largely because no effect is known to physics of any change brought about on a magnetic field due to the application of polaroids. The distribution of magnetic flux over both poles of a simple bar magnet was plotted using a *Squid Magnetometer*. This equipment is capable of measuring a change in magnetic field of the order of 10^{-11} of the earth's field and is currently the most sensitive magnetometer available. No change of any sort in the distribution of magnetic flux was noted when this investigation was carried out. The application of further polaroid filters over the magnetic pole under study again produced no change in the distribution of magnetic flux. Therefore the question as to what reticular energy is, if indeed it exists at all, remains open. However, in the author's view, and in the view of those practitioners making use of this in a therapeutic situation, there can be do doubt that a so-called polarized magnetic field is more therapeutically effective than a plain magnetic field. Perhaps further appropriate investigation may begin to reveal the mechanism of action of reticular energy and also the nature of this energy.

Electric, Magnetic, and Reticular Energy Nogier believes that three sorts of energy are present within the body, and he designates them electric, magnetic and reticular energy. Reticular energy has just been described. These names are derived from the ACR response to a battery (electric energy), to a magnet (magnetic energy) and to a polarized magnet (reticular energy). These energies are conceived as being present in layers, and they correlate with the concept of superficial, middle and deep tissue as described by Nogier. This concept of energy layers is in keeping with traditional Chinese ideas regarding the distribution of energy layers around the body; for example so-called wei energy was supposed to be present in the layer of the skin and just above it, and was supposed to act as defensive energy to incoming pathogenic energy. This concept was extended to include an understanding of disease in terms of its depth of penetration into the envelopes of energy which were thought to surround the body. This is illustrated graphically in Pien Chhio's encounter with the Chinese emperor (see Chapter 1, Part 1). This correlation with traditional Chinese ideas regarding energy, and also the fact that Nogier openly admits to no knowledge of traditional Chinese medicine, gives further weight to Nogier's observation of electric, magnetic and reticular energy.

In a normal right-handed individual, when the positive pole of a battery is brought towards the right ear, at approximately 6cm from the right ear a positive ACR should occur. If the same pole of the battery is brought up to the left ear in a right-handed person, then no positive ACR should be observed. Therefore Nogier designates the outer surface of the right ar of a right-handed person, the electric surface. Such an observation confirms that the electric energy is in order. This can be further checked by passing the positive pole of the battery across the forehead from the right side to the left side. In a right-handed individual a positive ACR should only be noted over the left side of the forehead. A gold filter consisting of a sheet of gold leaf may be used instead of the positive pole of a battery (positive = gold), and similar findings on the ACR should be obtained. The opposite situation pertains in a left-handed individual.

If a magnet is brought up to the right ear in a normal individual then no ACR should be obtained. If the same magnet is brought towards the left ear, then a positive ACR should be obtained, at approximately 6cm from the left ear. The pole which is brought up to the ear in this particular situation doesn't seem to matter. If the north pole of the magnet is passed over the forehead from the right to left in a normal right-handed individual a positive ACR should only be noted over the left forehead. If these findings are obtained, then magnetic energy is deemed to be normal, and as a consequence of these findings the outer surface of the left ear in a right-handed individual is termed the magnetic surface.

If a polarized magnet, that is a bar magnet with one or more polaroid sheets applied to either pole is brought towards the right ear of a right-handed individual, then no positive ACR should be obtained. The same findings should be obtained if the polarized magnet is brought up to the left ear. If the north pole of a polarized magnet is passed over the forehead from the right side to the left side, in a normal right-handed individual a positive ACR should be noted over the left forehead only. The opposite pertains in the case of a left-handed individual. If these findings are obtained, then it is assumed that reticular energy is in normal distribution. Nogier considers that the reserves of these energies, particularly the reserves of electrical energy that a patient should have, are important with regard to his response to disease, and in order to detect reserves of electric energy, which from a practical point of view is the most important reserve energy, the same procedure can be carried out. In other words, the positive pole of a battery is brought up to the right ear or a gold leaf filter is brought up to the right ear with the seven colour programme filter placed on sympathetic skin. If a positive ACR is obtained at the same distance from the right ear as was obtained without the seven colour filter on sympathetic skin the patient's reserves of electrical energy can be assumed to be normal. If on placing the seven colour programme filter on the forearm and the distance at which a positive ACR is obtained with either a gold filter or the positive pole of a battery from the patient's dominant ear is reduced, then the patient can be assumed to have poor reserves of electric energy.

This is taken as indicating that a focus of some sort is present, such as a tooth or a scar. Therefore, in order to help the patient, a search for a focus should be carried out; this can be done using auricular medicine, but in the author's view electro-acupuncture according to Voll is a more accurate way of locating a focus. So, the diagnostic procedure outlined above for detecting reserves of energy is a useful procedure from the point of view of getting the patient better, even though the explanation implied may be far from correct. The above concepts must be looked upon in terms of practical working concepts rather than as literally referring in a scientific sense to these so-called energies.

The Three Phases in the Ear Nogier describes, as well as the classical organization of the homunculus on the ear with the head on the lobule, the spine along the anti-helix (in other words an

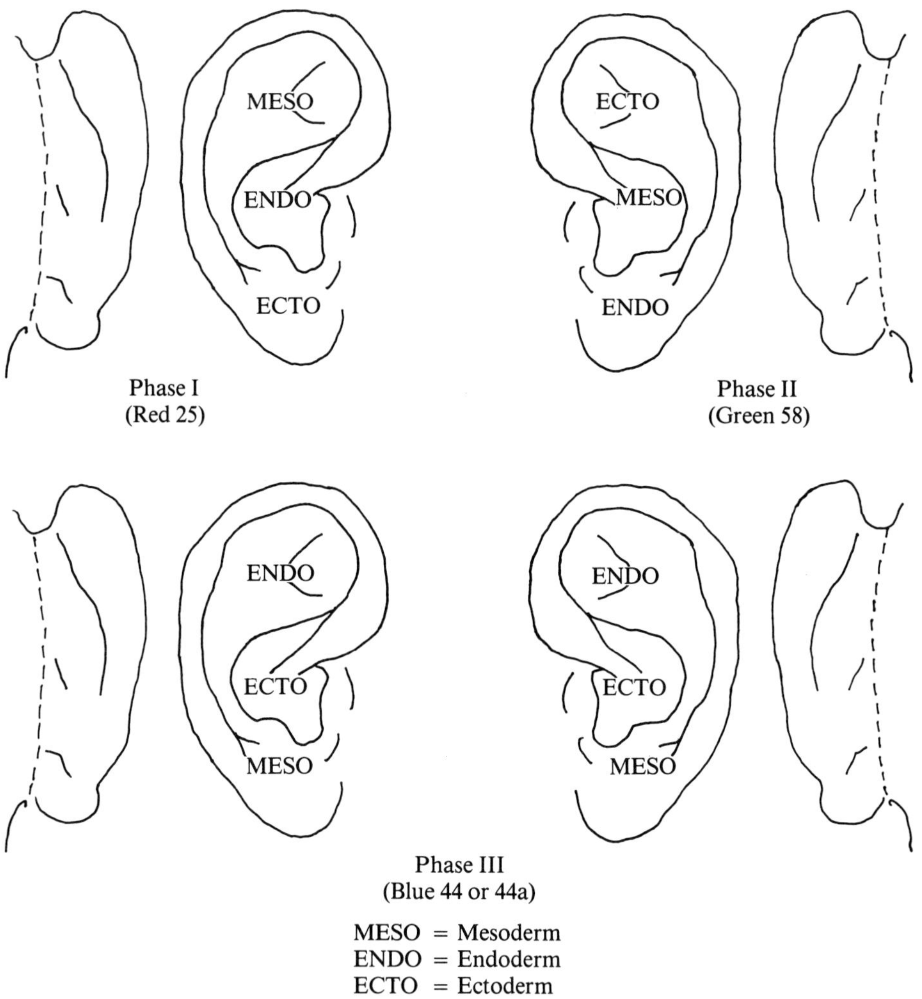

Figure 118.   Organization of the three embryological layers (endoderm, mesoderm and ectoderm) on the auricle in the three phases (after Nogier).

upside down foetus), two other possible localizations; these are termed 'phases'. The classical localization is designated Phase 1. In Phase 2 the head is present in the upper part of the ear, the limbs in the concha, and the viscera on the lobule; in other words the foetus is the rightway up in Phase 2.

Both Phases 1 and 2 are regarded as normal representations and are therefore not pathological.

The third phase is regarded as pathological. In Phase 3 the head is present in the concha, the limbs in the lobule, and the viscera in the upper part of the ear. In many ways this is reminiscent of the cycles of the law of the five elements; that is two physiological cycles (the Cheng and the K'o cycles), and one pathological cycle (the reverse of K'o cycle). Illustrations of these homunculi are shown in Figures 118, 119 and 120.

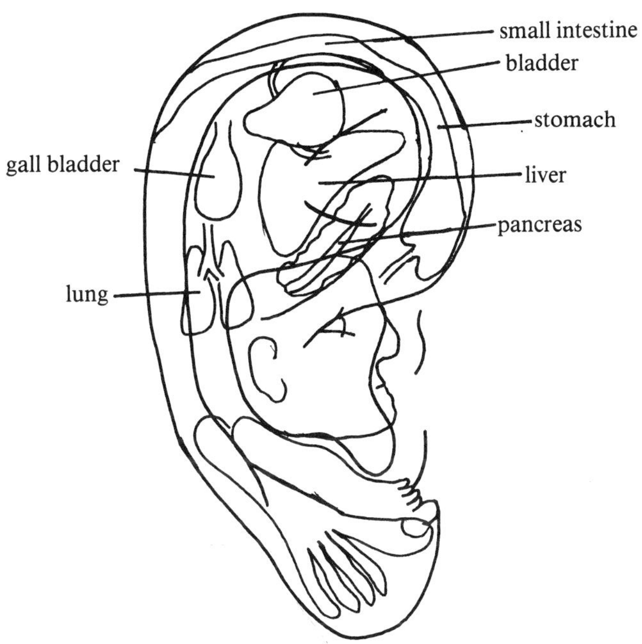

Figure 119. Somatotopic representation on the auricle in Phase III (pathological phase) (after Nogier).

In order to visualize what is happening in the three phases it is useful to imagine that in the first classical localization, mesodermal structures are represented in the upper part of the ear between the helix and the anti-helix, endodermal structures are represented in the concha, and ectodermal structures are represented in the lobule. In Phase 2, mesodermal structures are represented in the concha, ectodermal structures represented in the area between the anti-helix and the helix and endodermal structures are represented in the lobule. Then in Phase 3 ectodermal structures are represented in the concha; endodermal structures are represented in the area between the helix and anti-helix, and mesodermal structures are represented in the lobule. This is illustrated in Figure 118.

In Phase 2, the sequence of frequencies of the seven zones of the ear is reversed;

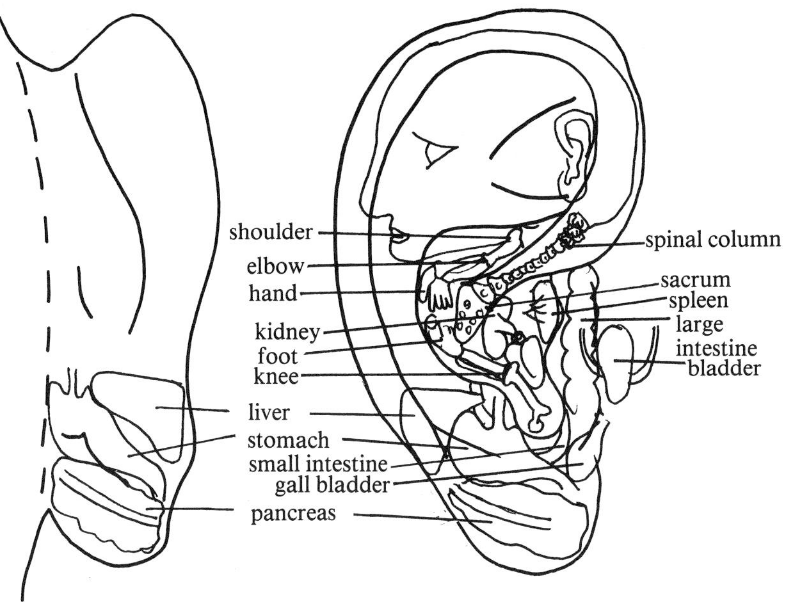

Figure 120. Somatotopic representation on the auricle in Phase II (after Nogier).

this is termed by Nogier as 'frequency inversion'; in other words, in Phase 2, zone C in the classical localization resonates as zone E, and zone B resonates at F frequency. The only zone to remain with its original resonance is zone D.

A particular colour filter has been found to correspond to each phase. Red Kodak Wratten Filter No. 25 corresponds to Phase 1; Green Kodak Wratten Filter No. 58 corresponds to Phase 2; Blue Kodak Wratten Filter No. 44 (or 44a as this is a very similar filter) corresponds to Phase 3. In the normal situation, Filter 58 brought towards the right ear of a right-handed individual should give a positive ACR at approximately 6cm from the ear; in other words, exactly the same as when a gold filter or a positive pole of the battery is brought up to the right ear when detecting normal electric energy, therefore electric energy is thought to correspond to Phase 2.

When Filter 58 is brought up to the non-dominant ear, no ACR should be noted at 6cm but one or two ACRs may be noted with the green filter approximately 1 or 2cm from the non-dominant ear. The opposite situation occurs in a left-handed individual. By inference, this means that Phase 2 representation of the homunculus is present on the dominant ear, and this has practical implications when searching for pathological points. However, it doesn't explain as to why good results can be obtained when treating as for the classical homunculus with the upside down foetus present on the dominant ear. Various explanations have been given for this, but unfortunately none are satisfactory. In the author's view, the present findings are probably not entirely correct, but they provide a practical working basis on which to achieve better clinical results, and should be used as such.

There is an unfortunate tendency among the various schools of acupuncture to regard their explanations for various phenomena as 'cut and dried', only to change

these again later when so-called 'new teachings' are either discovered, or in some
cases invented. If a Phase 1 filter, that is Red 25, is brought up to the dominant
ear (right ear for the right-handed individual) then no positive ACR should be
obtained at 6cm and possibly one or two ACRs may be obtained when this filter
is approximately 1cm from the dominant ear. If this filter is brought up to the non-
dominant ear, then a positive ACR should be noted 6cm from the non-dominant
ear in exactly the same way as the findings observed when a magnet is brought to
the non-dominant ear. Therefore magnetic energy corresponds to Phase 1.

Phase 1 also corresponds to the classical homunculus with the upside down foetus;
so by inference, the homunculus present on the non-dominant ear in the normal
situation is a classical representation.

Finally, if Filter 44 or 44a (either filter may be used) is brought up to either ear
in the normal individual, then no positive ACR should be obtained, and exactly
the same findings are observed with polarized magnets. Therefore Phase 3 is taken
as corresponding to reticular energy.

The above findings may all now be related in the following way:

Phase 1
A classical representation on the ear = Filter Red 25 = magnetic energy =
superficial tissue.

Phase 2
A representation of the foetus the right way up = Filter Green 58 = electric energy,
and corresponds to the deep tissue.

Phase 3
A representation of the foetus with the head in the concha and this representation
is regarded as being abnormal = Filter Blue 44 or Blue 44a = reticular energy and
corresponds to the middle tissue.

The concept of laterality has been mentioned earlier and is also applied to these
three energies. The concept of laterality involves more than right and left-
handedness. Nogier applies the concept of laterality in terms of energy balance in
the body. This concept was recognized by the ancient Chinese, and was partly what
yin and yang sought to explain. In classical acupuncture the closest concept relating
to Nogier's idea of energy distribution in the body, which he terms 'laterality',
concerns the so-called eight extra meridians, sometimes called 'marvellous vessels'
perhaps because of the often remarkable beneficial effect obtained if they are used
correctly.

The application of the eight extra meridians in classical acupuncture has been
more popular among European practitioners of acupuncture than among their
Chinese counterparts. The best review of the extra meridians is by Bierlaire.[3] In
simple terms, the eight extra meridians are supposed to mark boundaries between
energetic areas in the body, in that the body is divided into four quadrants, divided
from right to left by the anterior and posterior midline (the Renmo and the Dumo
respectively), another division running down the side of the body, dividing energetic
areas at the front from the back, and lastly, a line running round the middle of the

body, the so-called 'belt' channel (Dai mai). The ability to use these eight extra meridians competently has been restricted to practitioners with a clear understanding of energy balance. However, the results obtained from their treatment, if they are correctly chosen, are often remarkable, explaining their alternative name of the eight marvellous vessels. They are the exact counterpart of Nogier's concept of laterality. This concept is about energy balance in the body, and if that energy distribution is corrected, then health will often be restored. This therefore means that the concept of laterality as outlined here is of fundamental therapeutic significance. The understanding of the eight extra meridians and their use is a complicated procedure, but is recommended to all practitioners who consider their classical Chinese acupuncture to be at a sophisticated level. Nogier's concept of laterality is a simpler idea in therapeutic terms, Nogier applies the same concept to the so-called 'electric, magnetic and reticular energy' in that these ought also to be distributed from the right to the left side in a balanced fashion.

Detection of Disordered Electric, Magnetic and Reticular Laterality

In order to detect abnormal electric laterality a gold filter is brought up to the right ear. If no ACR is noted at 6cm but noted perhaps 1 or 2cm from the ear, then electric laterality is disordered, or alternatively, a gold filter can be passed from the right to left side of the forehead, and in a right-handed individual, a positive ACR should only be obtained over the left forehead. This test can also be carried out with the positive side of a battery.

In order to detect disordered magnetic laterality, the north pole of a magnet is passed from the right to the left side of the forehead. In a right-handed individual, a positive ACR should only be noted over the left side of the forehead. If this is not so, then magnetic laterality is disordered.

Lastly, for reticular laterality, a polarized magnet is passed from the right side of the forehead to the left side. Again a positive ACR should only be noted over the left side of the forehead in a right-handed individual. If this is not so, then reticular laterality is disordered.

If any or all of the above energies are found to be disordered in terms of laterality, then correction should be carried out before treatment begins. If this is done, then treatment is more likely to be successful. Correction of laterality itself can often relieve a difficult problem without any further theapeutic interference; this indeed is a remarkable finding and underlines the importance of the concept of laterality looked at in terms of energy distribution.

Methods for Correcting Disordered Electric, Magnetic, and Reticular Laterality

In order to correct disordered electric laterality the *Therapuncteur EMS.20* can be used with the so-called 'captors' (spring clips) connected to each ear, with the apparatus connected as shown in Figure 109. For a right-handed patient, the negative spring clip should be applied to the lobe of the right ear, and the positive spring clip should be applied to the lobe of the left ear. The positive spring clip should be the one which is connected to the red output from the *EMS.20*. The positive and negative buttons of the *EMS.20* should be depressed and the frequency U switched through on the apparatus. This direct current should be allowed to pass for approximately two minutes. The patient will feel nothing from this. After having carried this out electric laterality should be checked using either a positive pole of a battery or a gold leaf filter. If it is correct, then the procedure has corrected this disturbance of electric laterality.

For those practitioners without the *Therapuncteur EMS.20* apparatus, a simple piece of equipment can be made by connecting up two spring clips with electrically conductive jaws, connecting one to each pole of a 9 volt battery. These are then applied to the ear in exactly the same way as with the *EMS.20* with the negative clip applied on the right ear lobe of the right-handed person, and the positive clip onto the left ear lobe. Some electrode gel rubbed over the jaws of the spring clips will facilitate the passage of a current. With this arrangement the spring clips should be left on for twice as long as with the *EMS.20*, but generally this corrects disordered electric laterality.

In order to correct disordered magnetic laterality, a good rule of thumb is to use the *Theramagnetic-P*, having first removed the polaroid ear pieces as shown in Figure 114 with the south pole at the right ear, and the north pole at the left ear. This magnetic field should be passed for approximately two minutes, and then further tests should be carried out to see if this has corrected the magnetic laterality. In most cases it will have done so.

In order to correct reticular laterality a polaroid *Theramagnetic* is used, but this time the poles are reversed. The north pole is placed opposite the right ear, and the south pole is placed opposite the left ear. This magnetic field should be passed for approximately two minutes, and then reticular laterality re-checked.

These methods for the correction of magnetic and reticular laterality represent the consensus of opinion, and the official teaching from the school of auricular medicine. In the author's view giving a rule of thumb such as this is effectively the same as giving prescriptions for correction of the eight extra meridians in classical acupuncture. This is not a tenable concept, as each patient may require different needles in order to correct the extra meridians. This, in the author's view, also applies to disordered laterality, and in practice the author has found this to apply particularly to the correction of magnetic and reticular laterality. There, the ACR should be used to determine which pole and which strength of pole needs to be applied to each ear, using the techniques as described in the use of the *Theramagnetic* in Chapter 20.

It is not unusual to find that the magnetic laterality requires a different setting of the *Theramagnetic* in order to correct it, than does the reticular laterality in a patient whom both magnetic and reticular laterality are disturbed. Conversely, in some patients, one single setting of the poles of the *Theramagnetic* as determined by using the ACR is sufficient to correct both the magnetic and reticular laterality. This is not surprising as clearly each of the energies are related to one another.

In practice it is found that the polarized *Theramagnetic* generally is effective in correcting both the magnetic and reticular laterality, and that it is rare to have to remove the polaroid ear pieces.

As indicated above, in a normal individual, Phase 2 with the foetus the right way up (see Figure 120) should be present on the dominant ear (right ear of a right-handed individual). This is detected by a positive ACR with Green 58 at 6cm from the right ear, and Phase 1 with the classical upside down foetal representation should be present on the non-dominant ear, shown by a positive ACR; at 6cm from the non-

Detection of Phase Disorder on the Ear

dominant ear (left ear of a right-handed individual) with Red 25. If these findings are not made then there is a phase disorder. The most common finding is that over the dominant ear, instead of having a positive ACR with Green 58 at 6cm from the ear, no positive ACR is noted with Green, but a positive ACR is noted with Red 25 at 6cm from the dominant ear. This is described as Phase 1 parasitizing on Phase 2 on the dominant ear. The opposite situation may pertain on the left ear, in that Green 58 may be found giving a positive ACR at 6cm with Red 25 giving no ACR at all. This is described as Phase 2 parasitizing on Phase 1 on the non-dominant ear. The concept of parasites was outlined in Chapter 19 when describing the use of the *Theralaser*. A similar sort of concept is applied here.

Lastly, if Filter Blue 44 (or Blue 44a) gives a positive ACR at 6cm from either ear, or indeed at any distance from either ear, except when actually touching the ear, this indicates that Phase 3 is parasitizing onto whichever ear that a positive ACR with this filter is obtained. Before treatment is commenced these phases have to be corrected.

Procedure for Correcting Phases on the Ear The general principle applied is that the Phase which is parasitizing is used in order to detect the points responsible for this situation; in other words, if for example Phase 1 (Red 25) is parasitizing on Phase 2 on the right ear of a right-handed individual, then the method of correcting this is to use the turret lamp with Red 25 shining from the turret.

This colour which appears as a small round circle of red light projecting from the turret, should be passed over the right ear, and at one or more sites, a positive ACR will be noted. These sites should be marked with a felt tip pen and should be treated appropriately; in other words, they should then be detected with either a gold/silver or a positive/negative hammer to find the needle required in order to treat these pathological points.

Having corrected these points, and usually two points at the most are found responsible for this parasitizing, then the physical signs change back to normal, in that Green 58 over the dominant ear now gives a positive ACR at 6cm and Red 25 no longer gives a positive ACR at 6cm over the dominant ear but does so at 1cm.

It is interesting to carry out the following experiment:

If after having detected one or two points giving positive ACRs to passing the Red 25 colour, searching over the ear on which Phase 1 (Red 25) is parasitizing on Phase 2 (Green 58), then over these points a spring clip is applied, exactly the same as the spring clips used on the *Therapuncteur EMS.20*. If these are then left over these pathological points, and the filters are brought up again towards the ear it will be found that the physical signs have reverted to normal; in other words Green 58 now gives a positive ACR at 6cm. If one or both of these clips are removed then the physical signs revert to the abnormal situation.

The most likely explanation seems to be that these points are radiating some form of energy which is producing the disturbance, but when these points are closed over the situation reverts back to normal. In the author's view, this is a relevant finding, and leads one to suppose that acupuncture points are radiating energy of one sort or another. The nearest we have to visualizing this energy and to confirming this scientifically is outlined in detail in Dumitrescu's book, edited by the author.[4]

Another method of finding the so-called Phase parasites is, instead of using the turret lamp, the parasitizing colour (that is in the case of Phase 1 parasitizing on Phase 2), can be placed on the forearm. Therefore, filter Red 25 can be placed on the forearm, and the ear on which the parasite is occurring can then be searched directly by passing a Heine lamp closely over the surface of this ear, and finding the points which give a positive ACR. Similarly, for finding a phase parasite for Phase 3 parasitizing on either ear, instead of projecting Colour 44 from the turret lamp close against the ear, Filter 44 can be placed on the forearm and the appropriate ear searched with the Heine lamp. The same can be done for Phase 2 parasitizing on Phase 1, in this case Filter Green 58 will be used.

As stated earlier, Phase 1 and Phase 2 are regarded as normal phases; so when treating any pathological point, for example, a point representing the elbow on the ear, the point can be needled in both its representations, both Phase 1 and Phase 2, and it is more likely that a therapeutic result will be obtained. Those practitioners who have used auricular therapy for some time will have noted with some mystification, as indeed the author has, that often points 'light up' on the ear with the ACR using normal detection methods and these points appear to bear no relation to the site where the point would be expected to be, using the classical upside down foetal representation on the auricle. However, applying the idea of the second Phase to this makes sense of many more of these points. Therefore this is a useful application of the two phases. **Application of the Idea of Phases When Treating Pathological Points**

All of the above concepts may be summarized into a protocol which should be carried out prior to applying any treatment on a patient. This procotol includes all the new concepts outlined above, plus a number of concepts already mentioned. In order to be sure of obtaining maximal theapeutic efficiency this protocol should be gone through with each patient before using auricular medicine. With practice, this procotol should only take five or six minutes to run through:

1. Check for disordered laterality using the technique as outlined in Chapter 10 using B filter on the forearm and the pressure palpator. Abnormality here denotes a 'first rib' problem, which should be either manipulated or treated with a silver pin on the anti-helix on the point of the first rib and a gold pin on the helix, at the end of a radius drawn out from point zero through the point of the first rib.
2. Check for inversion, using Noradrenaline and Acetylcholine ampoules as outlined in Chapter 13. If inversion is found to be present, correct this using alternating polarized magnetic fields passed for two minutes across both ears.
3. Check for disordered electric, magnetic and reticular laterality. Correct as outlined in this chapter if found to be abnormal.
4. Check for good reserves of electric energy by putting the seven colour programme on the arm, and then checking to see whether the distance from the ear at which the gold leaf filter gives a positive ACR is reduced. If it is reduced by a distance of three or more centimetres, then the reserves of electric energy are low. This indicates a focus. The best way of searching for a focus and treating it is to use electro-acupuncture according to Voll, although auricular medicine can be used for this. For a tooth focus, simply search over the skin overlying the bottom or top jaw with a polaroid point detector, and treat any positive

unit as shown in Figure 122. The pulse wave is recorded by a pulsed ultrasound sensor mounted on a frame capable of moving in the X, Y and Z axes; this in turn is mounted within a plastic splint to fit around the forearm. A recording from the pulsed ultrasound sensor (Figures 123 and 124) is fed into a computer which has an integrating unit attached to it. The pulse shape is visualized on the oscilloscope, and the sweep speed of the X axis is increased until the wave shape which contains the ACR is focused on the screen. The recording obtained from the pulse sensor is shown in Figure 125 with an arrow pointing to the deflection referring to the ACR phenomenon within this pulse shape. The ACR pulse shape is shown in Figure 126 which shows a positive ACR. A negative ACR is shown in Figure 127. These wave shapes are fed via an integrating unit connected to the computer which records a high number for a positive ACR as shown in Figure 128 and a low number when showing a negative ACR; this is shown in Figure 129. Both the high and low numbers on the integrating unit, that is above and below the central midline measurement which is taken as zero, were taken at the same time as the positive and negative ACR wave shapes shown in Figures 126 and 127.

Navach has also isolated a number of other phenomena within the pulse; two particularly corresponding to sympathetic and parasympathetic waves. Navach claims that these particular wave shapes can be influenced by stimulation of indwelling electrodes to specific nuclei of the thalamus, this work having been carried out on experimental animals. All of the above work was presented at the Eighth German/Latin Congress on Acupuncture and Auricular medicine, Lyon, France, in September 1981.

Navach regards the ACR recording device as being useful in a clinical situation, as well as being important from a research point of view. This is possibly open to

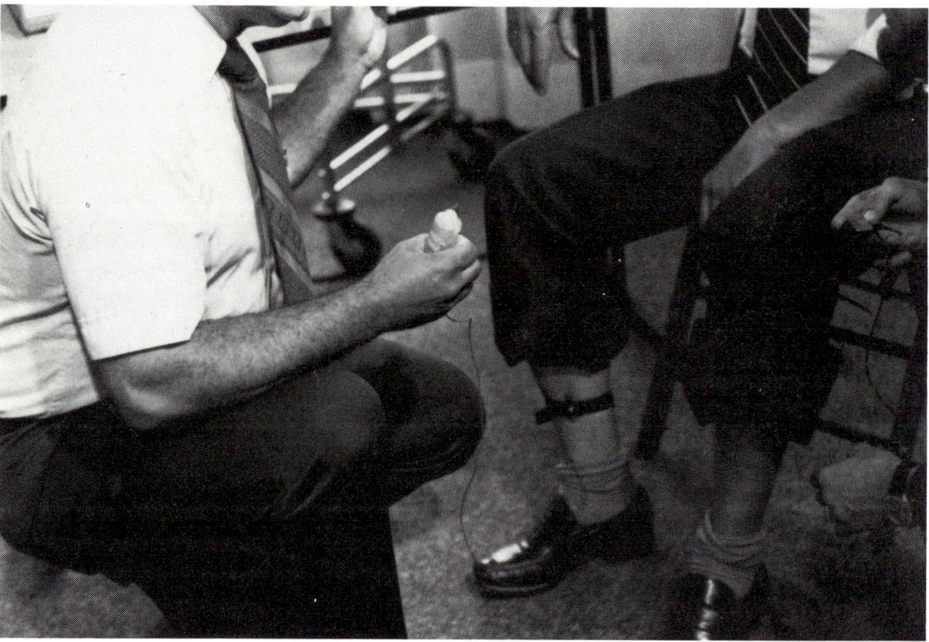

Figure 122.   Earthing the patient to the earthing unit.

question, as the equipment is expensive and includes a sophisticated computer. It remains a major contribution to the field of auricular therapy in particular, and medicine in general, and provides the first device capable of recording the ACR.

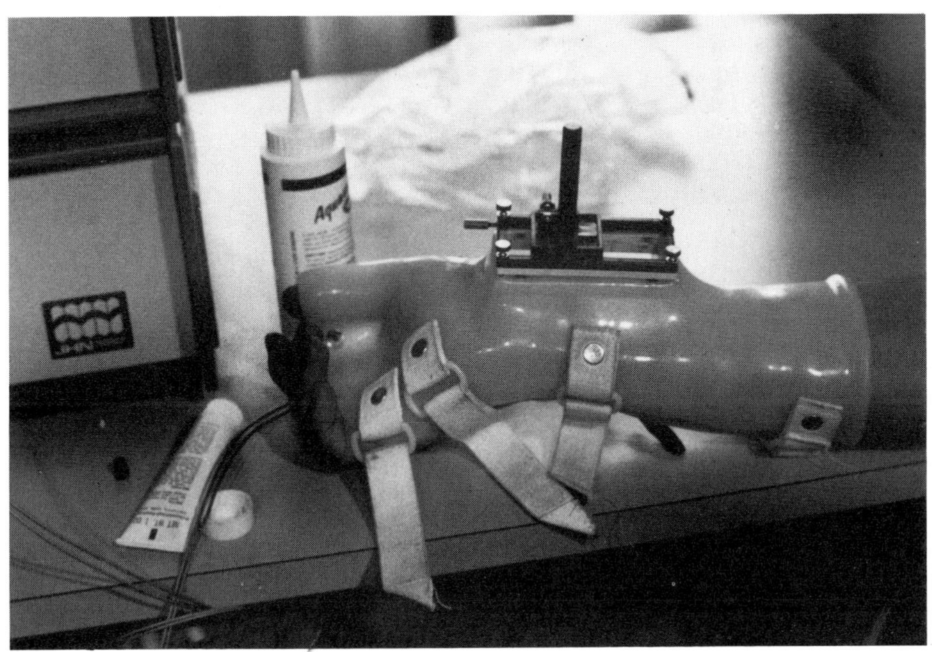

Figure 123. Pulsed ultrasound sensor mounted in a plastic splint.

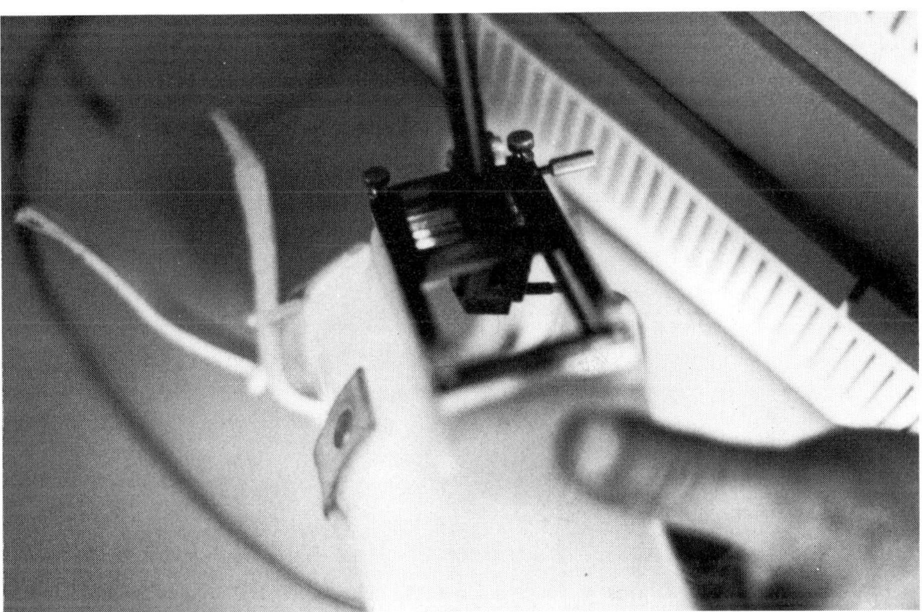

Figure 124. Close-up view of ultrasound sensor.

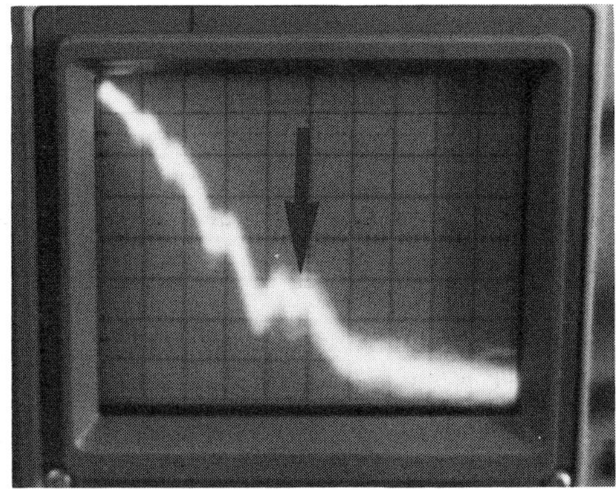

Figure 125. Recording obtained from pulse. Arrow points to area in recording which contains the ACR.

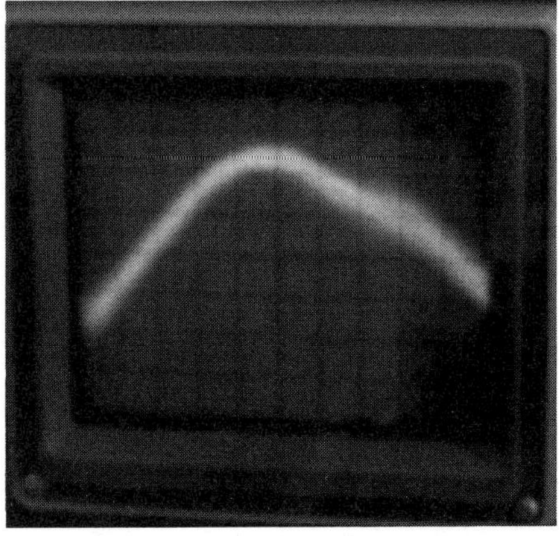

Figure 126. A positive ACR.

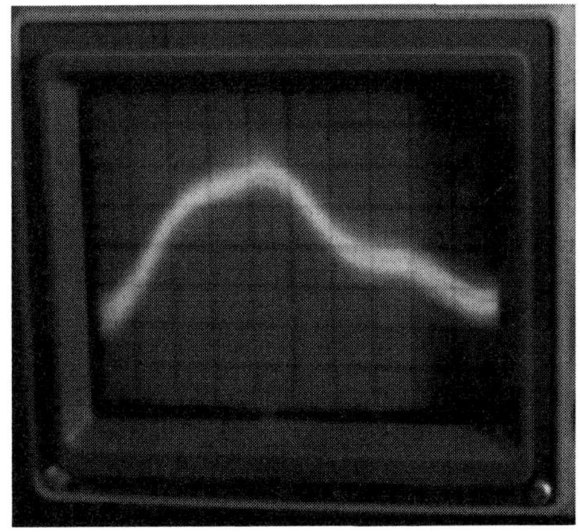

Figure 127. A negative ACR.

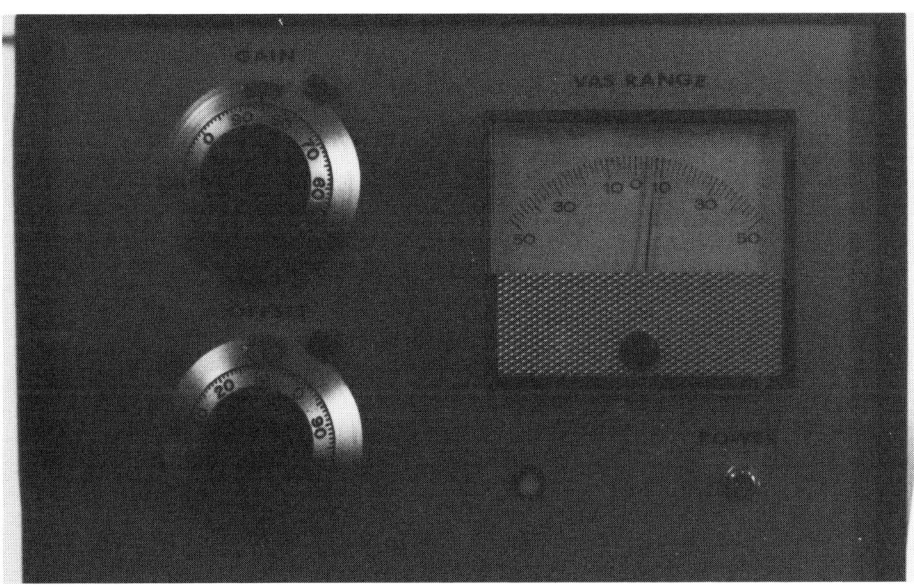

Figure 128.   A deflection to the right of the integrating unit signifying a negative ACR.

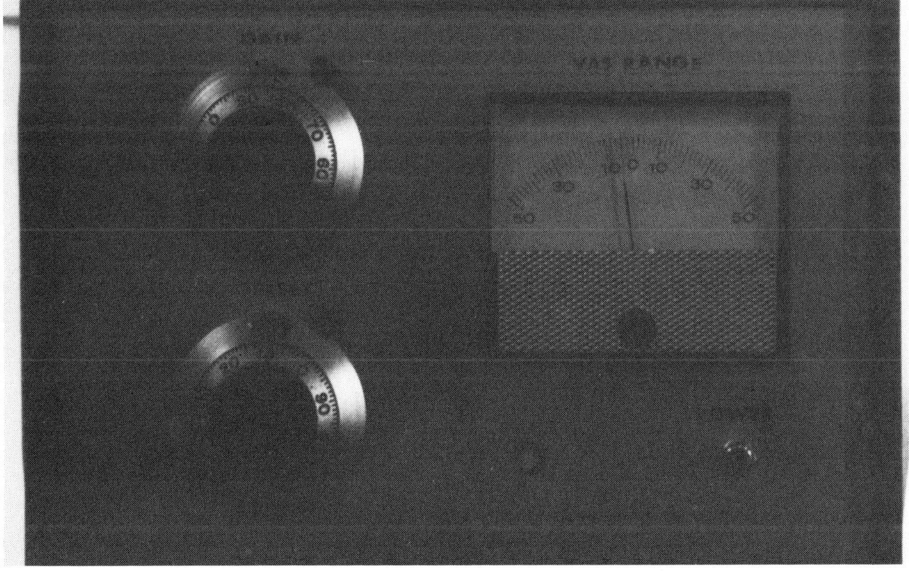

Figure 129.   A deflection to the left of the integrating unit signifying a positive ACR.

APPENDIX II

Equipment Required for Auricular Therapy	Pressure palpator (110 grams per square centimetre). Rubber earstamp. Semi-permanent ear needles. 1″ or ½″ Stainless Steel 30 gauge acupuncture needles. Chinese earpress needles. *Punctoscope* or a *Diascope*.

Equipment Required for Auricular Medicine

Heine light.

Gold and silver ear acupuncture needles — the rigid variety of these needles is recommended.

Set of seven colour filters, plus a colour programme consisting of 1 colour from each of the seven frequency zones of the ear.

Black/White hammer.

Positive/Negative hammer.

Gold/Silver hammer (optional).

Equipment Required for Advanced Auricular Medicine

Colour filters Green 58, Blue 44 and Red 25 (Filter E which is Blue 44, and Filter B which is Red 25 may be used. However, Green 58 will have to be obtained separately).

Gold filter consisting of a sheet of gold leaf.

Magnetic filter and a polarized magnetic filter.

Sheet of polaroid.

Theramagetic-P.

Theralaser DT.

Therapuncteur EMS.20.

Appropriate drug and food filters as required.

The majority of the above equipment is manufactured by Sedatelec, 135 Route Neuve, 39540 Irigny, France.

Drug and food filters are available from The Centre for the Study of Alternative Therapies, 51 Bedford Place, Southampton SO1 2DG, England.

German Academy for Auricular Medicine, 3904 Bronson Boulevard, Kalamazoo, Michigan 49008, U.S.A.

Chapter 15 1. Becker, R. O. 'Electromagnetic Forces and Life Processes'. *Technology Review*. M.I.T. Press, Cambridge, Massachusetts, U.S.A., 1972.
2. Becker, R. O. 'The Bioelectric Field Pattern in the Salamander I.R.E.' *Transactions on Medical Electronics*, 7 (1960), 202-208.
3. Becker, R. O. 'The Neural Semi-conduction Control System and its Interaction with Applied Electrical Current and Magnetic Fields'. Proceedings of the Eleventh International Congress of Radiology. Series 105, 1753-1759.

Chapter 16 1. Huneke, F. *Das Sekunden Phaenomen*. Haug Verlag, Heidelberg, West Germany, 1961.
2. Huneke, W. *Impletol Therapie*. Hippokrates Verlag, Stuttgart, West Germany, 1953.
3. Huneke, F. *Frankheit und Heilhung Anders Gesehen*. Tenth Edition. Staufen-Verlag, Kamplitfort, West Germany, 1959.

Chapter 17 1. Rinkel, H. J. Randolph, T. G. and Zeller, M. *Food Allergy*. Charles C. Thomas, Springfield, Illinois, U.S.A., 1951.
2. Miller, J. B. *Provocative Testing and Injection Therapy*. Charles C. Thomas, Springfield, Illinois, U.S.A., 1972.

Chapter 18 1. Konig, H. L. *Bio-information — Electrophysical Aspects of Electro and Magnetic Bio-information*. Urban and Schwarzenberg, Balitmore, U.S.A., 1979.
2. Pressman, A. S. *Electromagnetic Fields and Life*. (Translated from Russian by Sinclair, F. L., Edited by Brown, A. F.). Plenum Press, New York, U.S.A., 1970.
3. Persinger, A. M. *E.L.F. and V.L.F. Electromagnetic Field Effects*. Plenum Press, New York, U.S.A., 1974.
4. Sheppard, A. R. and Eisenbud, M. *Biological Effects of Electromagnetic Fields of Extremely Low Frequency*. New York University Press, New York, U.S.A., 1977.
5. Bassett, C.A.L. *Pulsing Electromagnetic Fields: A New Approach to Surgical Problems in Metabolic Surgery*. Edited by Buchwald, H. and Varco, R. L., 1978, 255-305.
6. Addington, C. et al. 'Biological Effects of Microwave Energy at 200mc' in *Biological Effects of Microwave Radiation* Vol. 1. Plenum Press, New York, U.S.A., 1978, 177.
7. Deichmann, W. 'Factors That Influence the Biological Effects of Microwave Radiation'. *Ind. Med. Surg.* 30 (1961), 264.
8. Schumann, W. O. and Konig, H. L. 'Atmospherics Geringster Frequenzen' *Naturwissens Chaften*, 41 (1954), 183-184.

9. Wiener, N. 'New Chapters in Cybernetics' (Translation from Russian), 1963.
10. Porkert, M. *The Theoretical Foundations of Chinese medicine*. M.I.T. Press, Cambridge, Massachusetts, U.S.A., 1974.
11. Becker, R. O. Reichmanis, M., Marino, A. A. and Spadaro, J. A. 'Electrophysiological Correlates of Acupuncture Points and Meridians'. *Psychoenergetic Systems* I (1976), 105-112.
12. Dumitrescu, I. F., translated from Rumanian by Galia, C. A. and edited by Kenyon, J. N. *Electrographic Imaging in Medicine and Biology*. Neville Spearman, Sudbury, Suffolk, 1983.
13. Leading article (author's name not supplied) 'Electromagnetism and Bone'. *Lancet* (April 1981), 815-816.

Chapter 19

1. Bischko, J. 'Studies in Therapeutic Effect of Laser Radiation in Classical Acupuncture'. Medicina Alternativa Congress, Amsterdam, Holland, 1980.
2. Pothman, W. 'Therapeutic Results From the Use of Lasers on Classical Acupuncture Points on Children'. Medicina Alternativa Congress, Amsterdam, Holland.
3. Mester, E. 'Klinische Unterschungen Uber die Wirkung van Laserstrahlen, Alf D, Wundheilung'. *Panmin. Med.* 13 (1971), 538.
4. Casper, K. H. 'Laser — Reiztherapie'. *Phis. Med. u. Rehab.* 9 (1977), 426, 455.

Chapter 20

1. Fichtner, N. *M.F. Therapy — Equipment and Operating in Practice*. Elec., Wiesbaden, West Germany.

Chapter 21

1. Rouxeville, Y. 'Thermometrie et Champs Magnetiques'. Eighth German/Latin Acupuncture and Auricular Therapy Congress, Lyon, France, September 1981.
2. Melville, D. and Lewith, G. T. Personal communication, 1980.
3. Bierlaire, J. 'Ontogenese des 8, Vaisseaux et des 12 Meridiens d'Acupuncture'. Seventh World Congress of the W.U.A.S.S., Florence, Italy. (An English translation of this text is available from the author on request.)
4. Dumitrescu, I. F., translated from Rumanian by Galia, C. A. and edited by Kenyon, J. N. *Electrographic Imaging in Medicine and Biology*. Neville Spearman, Sudbury, Suffolk, 1983.

selection of organ preparations available than any homoeopathic pharmacy to date. If the EAV practitioner is going to treat degenerative conditions using EAV, then an adequate supply of organ preparations and viscum preparations is essential.)

Source of EAV Texts Easy Asia Books Ltd.
103 Camden High Street
London NW1 7JN

EAV Seminars
PO Box 297
Sebastopol
California 95472
USA

Courses in EAV The Centre for the Study of Alternative Therapies
51 Bedford Place
Southampton SO1 2DG
England

Dr Peter Madill
EAV Seminars
PO Box 297
Sebastopol
Valifornia
95472
USA

INDEX

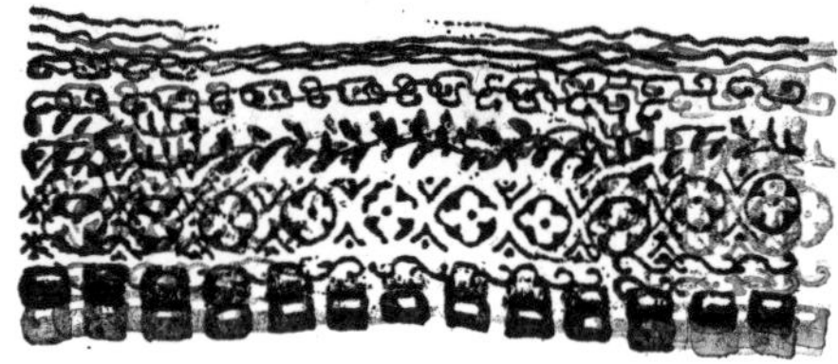